KOMBUCHA TEA

FOR YOUR HEALTH AND HEALING

THE MOST IN-DEPTH GUIDE

ALICK & MARI BARTHOLOMEW

GATEWAY BOOKS, BATH, UK

First published in 1998 by
GATEWAY BOOKS
The Hollies, Wellow,
Bath, BA2 8QJ, UK

© 1998 Alick & Mari Bartholomew

Distributed in the USA by
ACCESS PUBLISHERS NETWORK,
6893 Sullivan Rd, Grawn, MI 49637

Set in Palatino by
Synergie of Bristol
Printed and bound by
Redwood Books of Trowbridge

Cover design by Synergie of Bristol

British Library Cataloguing Data
A catalogue record for this book is
available from the British Library

ISBN 1 85860 049 9

Acknowledgements

The Kombucha Tea Network would never have got off the ground without the commitment and hard work of the coordinators who spread the good news and benefits of Kombucha therapy to their communities; our thanks to all of them.

This book would have been incomplete without the valuable feedback we have received from Kombucha brewers on the Network.

To Dr Neil Campbell-Brown and to Dr Monica Bryant for their advice and for checking the text, our appreciation of their support.

Especial thanks to Bob Macdonald of Pasadena whose gift of 'George', the progenitor of 200,000+ healthy cultures, was to seed healing, good health and self-empowerment to half a million people.

To Sue Shaw and her family for the photoshoot, and Tina Currie for her editorial work and advice, and to all at Gateway Books for helping to push the Kombucha boat out, our grateful appreciation.

Thanks finally to all colleagues, friends and family who have been understanding of our absence and have supported us while we were working on 'the book'.

Alick & Mari Bartholomew

CONTENTS

INTRODUCTION

It gives me great pleasure to recommend Mari and Alick Bartholomew's new comprehensive and objective book on Kombucha. Much hard work and research has resulted in gathering together the most up-to-date information on the subject.

After training in psychiatry, I elected to become a general practitioner in Cheshire and remained as senior partner in a large practice for thirty-two years. My previous experience helped me to treat my patients both for physical and emotional problems. This resulted in good rapport and empathy with them and undoubtedly assisted in their recoveries. Some resorted to alternative therapies which I accepted and supported if it contributed to their healing.

It was therefore interesting to me to be given a culture of Kombucha in 1981 from Hong Kong by Chinese patients. I believe that I was the only practitioner in the U.K. then to culture it and I used it for ten years. Having read a Chinese book on its therapeutic values, I was prepared to try it first on myself and on my family. My colleagues remained sceptical and biased, as were several laboratories who were not interested in analysing its potential therapeutic properties.

I found that it rapidly relieved arthritic pain and stiffness and that it cleared upper respiratory tract infections quickly. Because of my medical profession's prejudiced attitude, I had to be cautious in its use on patients, in case I breached my ethical code.

Over the next five years, with patients' consents, I introduced them to Kombucha and its use for relieving diseases. Resolution of leg ulceration, increase of energy and nail growth, clearing fungal skin infections, pigmentation of greying hair, improvement of gastro-intestinal disorders, were some of the main benefits that were found. On no occasion were adverse reactions reported. I also treated over many years a lady suffering from M.S., with beneficial results, leading to her quality of life being improved.

This comprehensive book will be of benefit to many people in their own homes and also to complementary health practitioners who are treating illnesses. I hope also that my own profession will read it and open their eyes to the full potential and benefits of this remarkable Kombucha health beverage.

To Mari and Alick, my thanks for starting the Kombucha Network and for their industry and faith in producing this book which can only further the search for the advancement of positive health.

Neil Campbell-Brown, MBChB

Note: Dr Campbell-Brown recommends that those with a diagnosable medical condition should seek the advice of a qualified medical practitioner before commencing Kobucha therapy.

CHAPTER I

THE STORY OF THE KOMBUCHA TEA NETWORK

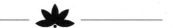

Why a Network?

When we picked up our first Kombucha fungus in June 1993 in Pasadena we had a vision - of hundreds of thousands of people in Britain being helped with all kinds of illnesses and health problems. That this has actually been fulfilled within three years is both exciting and very rewarding. We believe in networks. They are the way of the future and help to build supportive communities. Neither of us had started one before; it turned out not to be difficult, because we were supported by wonderful people who had discovered for themselves the remarkable properties of Kombucha tea and who also wanted to help as many people as possible discover this healing and nutritious drink. The Kombucha Tea Network was clearly an idea whose time had come!

Kombucha is made from sweetened tea into which of Kombucha fungus is placed and left to ferment in a warm place. It can taste like apple cider or a refreshing light wine, and you make it at home with a simple recipe at almost no cost. It prevents illness, and has excellent detoxifying and immune-enhancing qualities. Its origins are lost in history, but in the earliest records two thousand years ago it was known as 'the elixir of long life'.

Kombucha tea was known in the East, and found its way across Russia in the 1800s, becoming widely established as a folk medicine in many rural communities. In the 1950s it surfaced dramatically when Soviet doctors discovered whole communities which had apparently been protected from dangerous environmental pollution by an ancient food and folk remedy. This was a nutritious drink called tea-kwass or Kombucha tea.

How the Kombucha Network Started

Alick's cousin Bob was brought up in Niagara Falls in New York State, in a part of that old industrial city which had a polluted water supply. One after another, various members of his family died from cancer, and he saw the writing on the wall. He moved to Southern California, and began a search for something that would protect his and his family's health. Kombucha brewing was becoming established on the West Coast at that time, having found its way there from the Far East.

It was a hot day when we visited Bob in Pasadena. He told us the story of his search and how much he had been helped, and he insisted we taste his home-made Kombucha tea. We could both feel the energy spreading through our bodies and became very interested in knowing more about it. We heard many amazing stories from Bob of health benefits derived from regularly drinking Kombucha. It was also the special feature of this interesting pancake-like fungus that fascinated us both. That is, its ability to reproduce itself every week, enabling spare cultures to be passed on to friends and family.

Both of us have had a serious interest in healing for many years, Alick through his work as a therapist at the Bristol Cancer Help Centre, and Mari as a shiatsu practitioner. We could see how networking Kombucha could allow people both to help themselves and to help friends and family to better health. In the USA the fungus was being sold for about $60 (£36) a time, but we felt that Kombucha was a gift from Nature to help cleanse, balance and strengthen our bodies and immune systems, and that it should be shared freely, as it has been done traditionally in the East. We thought what a remarkable opportunity it would be to pass on good health and goodwill in our own communities.

Bob gave us a sheet of instructions on how to make the Kombucha tea, and we set off, with 'George' (as we named it) in a large jar submerged in some of Bob's tea-brew. Mari was the only person from our flight back home to be stopped by the customs officials with her basket containing fruit and snacks - and 'George'. The inspector went through everything, and when he asked "what's that?" of the jar, he seemed to be satisfied with the quick retort that it was a food, and he waved us on. Because of this incident, the basket and George did not go through the X-ray machine. It is quite accurate to call Kombucha a food, so we were not out of order.

Once home, we followed Bob's instructions and recipe carefully for making the Kombucha tea. Soon George was submerged in a bowl of freshly-brewed sweetened tea with the liquid that George travelled in as a 'starter'. We then set about making a space in the airing cupboard so that the fermentation process could begin. Sure enough, after a week, we had an apple cider-like drink that was really pleasant, and another culture, called 'Georgina' this time (the last one to be named!) which had reproduced and grown on the surface of the bowl. We soon had a growing list of interested colleagues, friends and family all wanting a 'starter' culture. We found that people were very curious about it, especially after tasting a glass of Kombucha tea. The instructions we had been given were duplicated and passed on. As Kombucha spread, people began telephoning us constantly with lots of questions: about brewing, how to look after the fungus, how much to drink etc. It quickly became evident that Kombucha tea brewing and its usage raised more questions for people than our instruction sheet answered. Our home telephone became more and more a 'hot-line'.

The Need for a Good Handbook and Informed Research

Alick happened to see a review of a new book - *Kombucha: the Miracle Fungus* - in an Australian magazine. It was written by a German herbalist who was an expert on Kombucha and had promoted its therapeutic benefits. Kombucha was becoming as popular in Australia as it was in America. We obtained a copy and saw that it was a helpful and authoritative book. To make it internationally acceptable required some changes, so with Harald Tietze's co-operation, Alick, an independent publisher, brought out a revised edition in the Gateway Books publishing list. Without this handbook the Kombucha Network and its tens of thousands of people supplied with Kombucha cultures could not have got under way. Harald still successfully distributes his self-published edition for the Australian market, along with Kombucha starting cultures.

Over the years, with new printings, further information has been added to the text of Harald's book, making it one of the better basic guides to Kombucha brewing. The reason for embarking on our own Kombucha book is that we feel the time is now right for Kombucha to be taken more seriously and accepted by the orthodox and complementary health professionals and to lay the foundations of Kombucha tea as a holistic therapy. Following the work of Professor Enderlein and others, we have a better idea of why Kombucha is so effective with many immune-deficient illnesses. We also want to share information and experiences told to us by people on The Kombucha Network UK, and their feedback on how people have been helped by drinking Kombucha tea. We have also accumulated our own knowledge and experience of brewing and drinking Kombucha for over four years. We are also in contact with doctors and complementary health practitioners who have shared their own experiences of how Kombucha therapy has helped themselves, and their patients and clients.

The Threat to our Immune Systems

Our immune systems are under threat as never before; sometimes in ways that we feel 'the experts' are unaware of, or in ways that none of us quite understands sufficiently. Modern science is not adequate to the task. Indeed, it may be said that, by creating an inhospitable environment, our present science and technology are responsible for the increasing levels of hazard to public health all over the world. Do we really know what long-term ingestion of the chemicals added to our public water supplies do to our bodies or what the lasting effect of antibiotics and hormones routinely added to animal feed may be? What about the chemical additives in most processed foods and the pesticides or organo-phosphates sprayed on vegetables and fruit? Even if we minimise the risk of these by filtering our water and eating organic food, can we protect ourselves from increased levels of radioactivity in soils all over the world, from air pollution and from the rapidly increasing exposure to electro-magnetic stress which has become part of our age of new technologies?

In this book we shall try to understand how to take care of ourselves better and look at ways in which we can help our immune systems to cope with the enormous changes in our diet and our environment. The establishment of the first national Kombucha network was inspired by the awareness of new threats to our health, with increased incidence of cancers, arthritis, chronic allergies and, especially of new viral conditions like Chronic Fatigue Syndrome (ME). As conventional medicine has no remedies for these, the problems can only get much worse. We have a vision that the health of society could be transformed, both by a better understanding of what our bodies need for health, and by widely using Kombucha's extraordinary detoxifying and metabolic balancing qualities, which are like those of no other known product.

How the Kombucha Network Operates

The Network from the beginning has been a voluntary organisation. Mari found, through the many enquiries that came into the Kombucha post office box, certain people wanted to take part in networking and to provide cultures and information about making Kombucha tea at home. They too were convinced of its many benefits and saw the potential of helping other people towards better health. It soon became obvious from this new growing band of dedicated Kombucha coordinators who were both caring and enthusiastic people, who literally shone through the mist, that they would become fully committed and authoritative brewers and producers, dedicated to helping other people in their local area of the country.

Our plan was to pass on spare cultures at no cost. This remains the Network's principle, though Harald Tietze helped us to be realistic about our costs, pointing out how necessary it was to reimburse the coordinators' overheads. Little did we know just how valuable Harald's advice was to be when the media discovered Kombucha, and the resulting volume of enquiries has virtually taken over all the regional Kombucha coordinators' lives at times.

All areas of Britain and Ireland are now covered, and at the time of writing there are twenty coordinators, each with their own trusted band of Kombucha brewers producing healthy starting funguses, making available a recommended book as a guide and offering advice, if needed, to beginners.

The Quiet Revolution

The most remarkable revolution taking place in society today is not the demand for political or social change, but for individual autonomy. It is happening because people are *waking up*, as though from a deep sleep, and nowhere is this more evident than in the area of their health. It's not that we are giving up going to doctors, nor is it an issue of alternative medicine versus conventional. It is more that we are actually starting to choose doctors and therapists who won't just treat and fix us - but who will *empower us,* and guide us towards healing ourselves.

The evidence for this can be found in the huge recent growth of avidly-read self-help health columns in the popular press. It is also the fastest growing subject in popular books on the market today. One local doctors' surgery found that their new lending library with books of information on disease was unpopular, but when they changed the emphasis to self-empowerment, and included complementary therapies, there was a huge interest (*see* page 134). There is a growing awareness of the damage being done by some of medicine's 20th century 'wonder drugs', like the dogmatically over-prescribed antibiotics. More and more people are beginning to proclaim, "This is my body!" and seeking how they can now help themselves.

People who take initiatives like this tend to be those who will choose alternative therapies or who make good health a priority over, say, buying another item of fashion clothing or a car accessory. It is all a matter of what people feel is important. But the main problem is one of a very passive attitude towards health. Governments everywhere put their resources into treating illness rather than on preventing it occuring in the first place! Politicians are typically self-interested and have a short-term view. Yet it has been shown that[1] an investment of, say £1 million, in a well-conducted campaign to publicise the prevention of heart disease could easily save ten times that amount in the cost of treating it. All that is required is just a bit more imagination and common sense!

Prevention of illness and building public health standards depends on reducing the intake of foods that are bad for us and the chemicals that are poisoning us. There has to be much more awareness of the importance of nutrition, a subject which, surprisingly, in Britain has been not been part of medical students' education. There is far too little awareness of the connection between poor nutrition and illness, or of how the nutritional content of commercially produced vegetables and fruit has diminished considerably in the last 50 years with the advent of intensive agricultural methods and the use of chemicals.

Kombucha is therefore an answer to a prayer, and at almost no cost! It is a highly nutritious food drink. It is such an effective **metabolic balancer** (helping the various organs work together), **probiotic** (supporting the beneficial bacteria), **adaptogen** (balancing processes that get out of kilter) and **detoxifier** (*see* Glossary) that if it were widely and intelligently used, the health of the nation could be transformed. This will not be done by promoting Kombucha as a trendy new health craze, but by carefully building it as a therapy into our health-care systems, both at home and by recommendation through a health professional.

The Interest is Out There!

Interest in Kombucha among British newspapers and magazines has grown, especially following its success in the United States. The *New York Times* reported that there were three million brewers coast to coast. Articles in Britain started appearing initially in West Country papers. Then we had our first trial by fire on the Richard and Judy "This Morning" show on independent television. It was seen by millions of people, causing their switchboard to get jammed, and produced the first huge flurry of enquiries.

This became a flood when the national paper *The Daily Mail* featured a half page article. It followed up a few months later with a piece in its popular health section which produced eight thousand enquiries to the Kombucha Network. Because of the major interest this caused, *The Daily Mail* then went on to commission a more detailed article, again producing approximately another 8,000 enquiries. On the tail of this we had a *Sunday Times* newspaper article, features in many magazines and more television and radio appearances. In total we had to cope with over 30,000 inquiries in nine months. Our home became more like a post office sorting room and the Kombucha Tea Network coordinators did sterling work coping brilliantly with the pressure of supplying so many starter funguses and handbooks, and answering patiently more questions from beginners on brewing Kombucha.

Popularity Brings its Problems

It's hard to tell how many people are now practising Kombucha therapy. Enthusiasm for a new product often wanes, especially when some people find that they have to spend a little time and energy making it.

Anything new, these days, can become trendy. It took only one or two personalities like Barbra Streisand or Meg Ryan to announce that they drank Kombucha and had gained great benefit, to attract the many for whom fashion is life's driving force. We know that Kombucha, which has stood the test of 2,000 years constant and often revered use, does not need commercialisation by hype. We expect that the interest in Kombucha will stabilise and that sensationalism will subside. Many families and communities will naturally pass on the Kombucha culture with awareness of its many and varied health benefits; of cleansing their bodies, strengthening and building up their immunity. In these modern times we are becoming increasingly more vulnerable to environmental pollution and stress of one kind or another. Kombucha will come to play an important role in the health and strength of the nation, and become a part of life, maybe like the traditional 'cup of tea'!

The majority of people who want to start making Kombucha tea already have a health problem. Usually it is one which has not been greatly helped by conventional medicine, or where discomfort has been increased by the side-effects of prescription drugs. But many have also been impressed by how a friend or relative has been helped through taking Kombucha, and understand that one of its principal benefits is the overall improvement in body functioning.

Occupational Hazards

There were two main concerns which we faced in the Kombucha Tea Network. One was to dispel over-sensational claims for Kombucha's benefits. It was being described in some circles as a panacea for all ills, claiming to help cure every condition from ingrowing toenails to baldness! It is difficult, in a symptom-based medical system, for people not to expect a cure for their specific illness, rather than to look for an understanding of the underlying causes of that illness or imbalance. The human body is a wonderfully wise organism which is constantly seeking health and balance, but when it has been abused after many years (and even generations), it gradually breaks down. Through Kombucha therapy, and once it has been brought back to strength through detoxification, improved functioning and an enhanced immune system, the body can create the right conditions for its own natural mechanisms and healing to come into play. This is our perception, and one of the aims in writing this book is to promote a better understanding of this process of self-healing. We have the power in our own hands to heal ourselves, with a little help and wisdom from Nature. We can take charge of our health - body and mind - and become increasingly aware of what harms and weakens, and what heals and strengthens us.

Our other major concern was to foster a high standard of Kombucha tea brewing. Our original idea was to let the Network grow solely by encouraging any person who wanted to pass on cultures locally, thereby connecting people to each other. This, of course, does happen naturally, and is entirely appropriate. However, we found that not everyone who makes Kombucha produces healthy enough cultures. The reasons can vary from a wrong recipe or ingredients, inadequate warmth in fermentation or a failure to follow some of the basic golden rules of Kombucha brewing. We obviously can't check every Kombucha culture in the country that is passed on, but we can set a standard and take responsibility for ensuring that only healthy starter cultures and correct information originate from the Kombucha Tea Network and its coordinators.

Just as cuttings in the garden must be propagated from healthy plants, so you should begin your Kombucha brewing from a strong healthy 'mother' culture which will produce healthy new 'offspring'. In this way you can be assured of a good start in your Kombucha brewing life. Our main emphases are to encourage *safe* and *informed* brewing.

Encouraging Self-Empowerment

The Kombucha Tea Network is now like a big family of like-minded people who for the most part have found that Kombucha therapy has made a difference to their lives; in many cases significantly. A large proportion of people who have found that conventional treatments have not worked for their specific illness (sometimes even compounding their problems), have found great satisfaction, as well as relief from their suffering, by being able to take some responsibility for their own health by making and drinking Kombucha tea. Self-empowerment and taking responsibility are important tools for discovering more meaning, health, happiness and fulfilment in life, which is why we stress these in this book.

A growing number of people who are concerned about falling standards in public health and are worried about the effects of the many forms of pollution on their health, have found Kombucha to be a valuable asset in detoxification and in boosting their immune systems. As one gets older, especially if we have followed an imbalanced lifestyle, the metabolism becomes weaker, imbalances become more pronounced, and the deficiencies of modern allopathic medicine seem more obvious.

The most enthusiastic responses we have had to Kombucha have come from those people with difficult long-term illnesses and from older people. In addition, alarming numbers of young people are increasingly developing illnesses resulting from poor immune systems, such as eczema, allergies, Chronic Fatigue Syndrome (ME) etc. One of the advantages of Kombucha therapy is that it is available to everyone, regardless of age or economic resources. The good news is that this remarkable health beverage is very easy to make and is available to us all at very little cost.

We sincerely believe that to brew Kombucha tea successfully, people need to have as much information as possible. While it is very easy to make, some basic rules need to be followed. As everyone is different, individual reactions and improvements experienced from this healing beverage will vary greatly. With hundreds of thousands of people now brewing Kombucha in Britain, it is clear that our other vision of many people creating their own networks with their own family and friends, and in their local communities, is being realised. Soon, anyone who wants to obtain a starter culture will be able to do so quite easily, just as people in Russia, China or Japan have done for centuries.

From our first gift of a friendly fungus, we have successfully 'seeded' the British Isles and, indeed, many other countries too, to whom they have been sent.

WHAT IS KOMBUCHA?

Kombucha isn't really a fungus, far less a mushroom. Microbiologists insist it's more like a lichen. It is a symbiosis of bacteria and yeasts living together in a cellulose pancake-like culture, nourished by an infusion of sugar and tea. How this little chemical factory ever got started is a mystery that we'll never solve, because it is lost in the mists of time. Eastern tradition says that originally it came from the sea, and interestingly what the Japanese call 'Kumbu' is in fact a sea algae that still exists in a natural environment. Our Kombucha has been domesticated for thousands of years.

Tea is a herb as old as Kombucha's origin, but sugar is a modern processed food. Its predecessor in the fermentation process may have been a kind of grain malt, containing natural sugars.

In recent years, this extraordinary ancient remedy has enjoyed an upsurge of renewed interest - particularly in Australia, the USA and, most recently, the UK. This book sets out to explain what has made Kombucha one of the most popular and effective complementary health therapies if our time.

And What to Call It? In 'Kombucha circles' Kombucha is called either a 'fungus' or a 'culture' (mushroom is quite incorrect), so we shall alternate between these two terms throughout the book.

REFERENCE

1   BBC News, 9 Nov. 1997.

CHAPTER 2

THE HISTORY OF KOMBUCHA

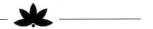

Two Thousand Years in the Far East

The earliest reference to the Kombucha tea-fungus was found by Pastor Weidenger, a missionary in Taiwan, to date over two thousand years ago to the Tsin Dynasty of the Chinese Empire in 221BC[1]. It was then known as the 'elixir of long life' or 'the Divine Tsche' (word for tea). Later it apparently found its way into Korea, for it was in AD14 that a Korean medicine man called Kombu used it to treat the Japanese Emperor Inkyo's disorders.[2] Pastor Weidenger's research suggests that the name derives from Kombu and the Chinese word for tea - 'ch'a', hence Kombucha. The German author Günther Frank, however, holds that the name derives from the Japanese word 'kombu' for seaweed - thus seaweed tea.[3]

Vinegars like acetic acid enjoyed widespread use for their refreshing qualities as far back as[4] 3000 years ago (see Chapter 12). During the following millennium the exceptional nutritional value of communities of yeasts and bacteria were discovered in health-promoting fermented drinks and food. An ancient relative of these is the Kombucha culture which has had a consistently favourable record for promoting good health for two thousand years. Kombucha, like herbalism, was part of natural medicine that formed part of everyday life up until relatively recent times, and now thankfully is beginning to make a come-back.

There was a tradition among Japanese warriors in mediaeval times to carry Kombucha tea in their hip flasks into battle to give them greater energy. From Japan and China, the use of Kombucha travelled through southeast Asia, reaching the Philippines, Java and India. C. H. Gadd says that it became popular in Java because Islam prohibits alcohol. In the Philippines the culture is still sold as a sweetmeat. Harald Tietze lists 120 different names for Kombucha tea from many languages, which testifies to how widely Kombucha therapy has spread round the world.

A Russian Folk-Remedy

There seems to have been a long continuous use of Kombucha in Russia. In many rural communities it was established from mediaeval times as a folk remedy for health maintenance and to slow down aging. Thought to have originated in China, Kombucha was brought to the Baltic countries by Russian sailors by the beginning of this century, and its use spread widely through Eastern Europe before the first World War. The shortage of sugar and tea during the Second World War restricted the fermenting of Kombucha, but after the war it re-surfaced in Germany, Italy, France and Spain.

Kombucha was part of the folk medicine tradition in rural Russia, much of whose culture was untouched by Western medicine. So it is appropriate that the first serious modern institutional research was conducted in the Soviet Union. Günther Frank has published an account by a Russian doctor of some remarkable research done at the Russian Academy of Sciences and the Central Oncological Research Institute in Moscow.[5]

After the Second World War, the cancer rate in the Soviet Union was rising rapidly. Of great concern was the high frequency of cancers in areas of heavy metal and asbestos pollution within the Western Urals industrial region. The Soviet Academy of Sciences and the Moscow Central Institute for Oncological Research instigated a research project to collect information. Two districts had been identified where the pollution was more dangerous, with terrible effects on the trees and the fauna. Yet cancers among the residents were very few, and those that there were, were found only in people who had recently moved there. It transpired that in these two environmentally devastated areas there were communities which seemed to enjoy extraordinary good health. The research doctors eventually stumbled upon what they were looking for when they were offered an hospitable glass in a family's home and were told, "We all drink this". These communities were found to consume a fermented brew that they called 'tea-kvass' (or Kombucha tea). In spite of there being a higher consumption of alcohol and nicotine, the work morale was considerably higher than in other parts of the USSR. Alcoholics who consumed significant quantities of this brew showed little signs of inebriation. Drunkenness was almost unknown. Here was a beneficial and cheap folk beverage which kept them all well.

Political Opposition to Kombucha Research

The first to benefit from Kombucha's research was Josef Stalin who had an obsession about dying from cancer. Dr Benga, who arranged his treatment, was Jewish, and became the victim of a plot by jealous officials who used Stalin's antisemitism to accuse him of trying to poison Stalin with a dangerous fungus. The outcome was the famous 'Doctors' Trial' of 1953 which led to the discrediting of Kombucha therapy in the Soviet Union. Its use continued on the margins of civilisation. Indeed the Nobel prizewinning novelist Alexandr Solzhenitsyn wrote in his autobiography that it saved his life in the Siberian slave camps.[6]

This change in medical emphasis in the Soviet Union after 1953 resulted in its alienation from all forms of natural medicine which continued to be practised elsewhere, in particular in Germany. It followed, therefore, that the interest in Kombucha would shift from Russia to Germany in the 1950s.

Kombucha Spreads World-wide

Dr. V. Koehler's work with glucuronic acid (one of the principal consituents of Kombucha), with both trees and humans in the early 1960s was a breakthrough. He was followed by Dr. Rudolph Sklenar who pioneered treatments of cancer patients with Kombucha. In the 1970s the drinking of Kombucha tea became quite popular in Germany.

During the late 1950s Kombucha drinking became a fashion in Italian high society. Fads can end as quickly as they start, and it only took a malicious rumour about Kombucha that caused the interest in Kombucha brewing to die off for a time. Reports of the beneficial effects of drinking

Kombucha in Swiss scientific research a few years later was able to restore confidence in the tea-brew, so that it was soon again available in chemists' shops.

In the 1990s, Harald Tietze, a German-born herb grower in New South Wales, was mostly responsible for its popularity in Australia, where he runs a thriving natural health support network. Germany has a well-established tradition of natural medicine and most of the independent research in the last century has been conducted and written about in that country. In other western European countries the interest in Kombucha is cyclical, probably because it has been seen as a fad, and because so little was known about it at a medical level.

Individual Kombucha funguses were brought into the United States, as to many other countries, in the 1960s, but they were not publicised or networked. It was not until about 1990 that, largely thanks to its popularity with HIV sufferers, Kombucha tea started to be widely networked there, especially on the West Coast. In Britain, apart from isolated individual importations, its introduction began with the formation of the Kombucha Network in 1993.

The Naturopathic Interest in Kombucha

Interest in Kombucha in Russia and Germany was probably due to the fact that medical thinking there is more flexible than in most Western countries. Germany, indeed, has a long tradition in naturopathic medicine. In the USA and in Britain, there has been much more scepticism in conventional medical thinking towards Kombucha therapy (see Chapter 3).

The main interest in Kombucha has been among those people who feel that conventional medical practices are not successful with many chronic diseases, particularly those related to immmuno-deficiences. It is not surprising, therefore, that the holistic and naturopathic areas of medicine have been most receptive to Kombucha's health benefits.

With greater awareness of environmental pollution and stress factors, and the limitations of conventional therapies in countering them, the potent anti-toxic and immune-enhancing qualities of Kombucha are likely to be increasingly recognised and welcomed. Some authorities believe that our immune systems will come under greater stress from growing exposure to photon energies in the cosmic environment. The endocrine (immune) and haematological (blood) reactions in our bodies that are beginning to be monitored as a result of this, will be greatly aided by Kombucha's ability to balance our metabolic functions. We can therefore expect a wider orthodox acceptance and more general popular use of Kombucha therapy internationally in the coming decades.

REFERENCES

1   Tietze, Harald, *Kombucha - Miracle Fungus*, Gateway, 1995.

2   Fasching, Rosina, *Tea Fungus Kombucha*, Ennsthaler, 1987.

3   Frank, Günther, *Kombucha: Healthy Beverage and Natural Remedy from the Far East*. Ennsthaler, 1991.

4   Fasching, Rosina, *op. cit.*

5   Frank, Günther, *op. cit.*

6   Solzhenitsin, Alexandr, *The Cancer Ward*, Bodley Head, 1970.

CHAPTER 3

HOW DOES THE FUNGUS WORK?

Most people we talk to about Kombucha initially think it must be a kind of health tonic. They find the idea of 'Kombucha therapy' rather strange. When we looked at the other available books on Kombucha, we quickly saw that there was a need for a more in-depth book. We realised that we would also have to attempt what we felt no other book has done satisfactorily - to make a credible case for why Kombucha is so helpful with diseases like arthritis, eczema, high blood pressure, digestive disorders and cancer, to mention a few. If our modest efforts to explain 'how Kombucha works' encourages more serious research at the holistic microbiological level, we shall be delighted. Our understanding of the causes of disease is going through an enormous change, as we learn more about the inner ecology of the body. This will affect how medicine will be practised in the future, and it is exciting to realise that the way Kombucha works will be part of this new understanding.

The Germ Theory

For the last 150 years medical treatments have been based on the concept that the invasion of a particular pathogenic (disease-causing) micro-organism causes a specific disease. The germ theory, on which it is based, dates only from the mid-nineteenth century, and has led, a hundred years later, to the introduction of antibiotics whose purpose is to kill the offending microbes.

Antibiotic (anti-life) Therapy

The discovery and use of antibiotics has been hailed as the greatest medical breakthrough of the century. Indeed, it has undoubtedly saved many thousands of lives, and still has a valuable place in the control of life-threatening systems. However, an increasing number of problems have arisen from its widespread over-use, both for human treatment and as a standard animal food supplement. One is the increase of diseases caused by the treatments themselves (iatrogenic diseases), which cause a growing number of deaths, as well as complex side-effects. The second is that antibiotics can weaken the body's own immune system, which then makes it more difficult to fight off new germs and viruses. The third, and undoubtedly much more serious problem, is the emergence of bacterial strains which are resistant to antibiotics.

This problem has its parallel in the development of pest control and herbicides in industrial agriculture. They were hailed as a great breakthrough in agricultural science, but have not stopped the emergence in crops of new diseases that are much harder to control. These stem from the way in which the chemicals tend to kill both the natural predators and the bacteria in the soil that help to provide the plant with balanced nourishment and which are part of a self-sustaining ecosystem.

Follow Nature

Hippocrates (370-260BC), who lived in ancient Greece and who is usually regarded as the founder of modern medicine, practised a form of medicine which advocated working with the balancing power of Nature. He was an outspoken critic of the administration of drugs and of unnecessary meddling by the physician, believing very strongly that the body has a self-healing mechanism that must be aided in every way possible naturally to heal itself. Hippocrates instructed his students to follow Nature and to do no harm to their patients. All doctors, on graduation, swear to honour the Hippocratic Oath!

The oldest form of medicine, which is still practised successfully today, is herbalism. The use of the whole plant to assist human disorders has been the common denominator of healing for tens of thousands of years. Many modern pharmaceutical drugs are inevitably based on plant constituents, the difference being that individual parts of the plant are extracted and synthesised in the laboratory in order to counter specific symptoms. For example, the common drug aspirin, a pain killer and blood thinner, has the harmful side effect of causing stomach irritation and ulcers if over-used, whereas the whole plant Meadowsweet (*Filipendula ulmaria*), used in its natural state from which aspirin is derived is, in fact, *very beneficial to the stomach*, and is its main healing property. Since the pharmaceutical industry has become dependent on synthetic chemicals, their effectiveness in bringing healing to the whole system has been compromised, with side effects that are treated with further drugs, and so on.

Probiotics (Pro-life!) Therapy

In terms of modern medicine, the naturopathic or holistic approach in which the working of Kombucha can be seen, is called probiotics.[1] This means working with the microbiological life (pro=with; bios=life) rather than destroying the microbes which is the purpose of antibiotic therapy.

The probiotic case for Kombucha is that it encourages much healthier intestinal flora by introducing lactic acid-producing bacteria. These work in a similar way to acidophilus bacteria, the active ingredients in live yoghurt.

An old saying, 'healthy gut, healthy body,' puts it simply. The digestion is the physiological system that uses enzymes to break down complex food into simpler components which can be used by the body cells, its principal organs being the stomach and the small and large intestines. The acidity level of the gut is all-important, as is the health of its microbial flora. There are several hundred different species of bacteria in our intestines and there is abundant evidence that the intestinal flora plays a crucial role in the functioning of the whole body.

Bacteroides and Bifidobacteria

The bacteria in the intestines can be divided into two main types:[2] the less acid-forming bacteroides are responsible for the decaying matter in the colon; elderly people tend to have more gastric disorders; these stem from a

3low hydrochloric acid production in the stomach, creating more room for fungi and parasites to take hold; bacteroides are encouraged by a diet high in fats and proteins.

The more acidic ones, called bifidobacteria, are more beneficial because they produce essential organic acids, such as acetic, lactic and folic acids, which raise the acidity of the intestines, preventing invading pathogens from taking hold. In addition, by keeping down the bacteroides population, they discourage the putrefaction from becoming toxic. The bifidobacteria are favoured by a diet high in carbohydrate, fibre and lacto-vegetarian food and are more common in individuals who were breast-fed as babies.

Kombucha - a Nutritious Food

The Kombucha beverage should be regarded principally as a food unusually rich in nutritive properties, rather than just a health drink. As in yoghurt, the bacteria are a great source of nutrition, but in addition Kombucha has a wide range of organic acids, vitamins and enzymes that give it its extraordinary value. It contains the range of B vitamins, particularly B1, B2, B6 and B12, that provide the body with energy, help to process fats and proteins, and which are vital for the normal functioning of the nervous system. There is also Vitamin C which is a potent detoxifier, immune booster and enhancer of vitality.

Probiotic Organic Acids

There are two organic acids produced by Kombucha which encourage the activity of the resident bifidobacteria, thus restoring a healthy balance with the bacteroides:

Lactic acid which is essential for healthy digestive action (through its derivative lactobacilli) and for energy production by the liver, and is not found in the tissues of people with cancer.

Acetic acid which is an antiseptic and inhibitor of pathogenic (harmful) bacteria.[3]

Kombucha's Vital Organic Acids

Besides the lactic and acetic acids mentioned above, there are also other valuable organic acids produced by the Kombucha culture, some of which have a more direct effect on other organs[4]:

Glucuronic acid is normally produced by a healthy liver, is a powerful detoxifier and can readily be converted into glucosamines, the foundations of our skeletal system.

Usnic acid has selective antibiotic qualities which can partly deactivate viruses.

Citric acid is an antiascorbic.

Oxalic acid encourages the intercellular production of energy, and is a preservative.

Malic acid also helps the liver to detoxify.

Gluconic acid is a sugar product which can break down to caprylic acid to work symbiotically with -

Butyric acid (produced by the yeast) protects human cellular membranes, and combined with Gluconic acid which is produced by the bacteria, strengthens the walls of the gut in order to combat yeast infections such as candida.

Nucleic acids, like RNA and DNA, transmit information to the cells on how to perform correctly and regenerate.

A product of the oxidation process of glucose - glucuronic acid - is undoubtedly one of the more significant constituents of Kombucha. As a detoxifying agent, it has come into its own today, for it is one of the few agents that can cope with pollution from the products of the petroleum industry, including all the plastics, herbicides, pesticides and resins. It 'kidnaps' the phenols in the liver which are then eliminated easily by the kidneys. Another byproduct of glucuronic acid are the glucosamines, the structures associated with cartilage, collagen and the fluids which lubricate the joints. Collagen reduces wrinkles, while arthritis sufferers have their deficient cartilage and joint fluids replenished.

Amino acids, which are constituents of proteins, produce important enzymes, such as glutathione a powerful antioxidant which provides protection from alcohol and pollution, and which is depleted by drug regimes.

All Kombucha cultures differ, but produce similar effects!

The specific organic acids that are found in the Kombucha beverage will vary according to the proportion of bacteria to yeast cells, and to the particular species of each. It is undoubtedly true that, despite the variation of species of yeasts and bacteria found in Kombucha cultures all over the world and over time, amounting to different species types, the effect on the human body seems to be similar. This does not help the microbiologist whose discipline requires constituents to be identical in order to come to deductive conclusions about the efficacy of Kombucha for certain diseases or physical conditions. Medical herbalists are familiar with the idea that a whole family of plants provide 'a particular message' or a specific healing property, no matter what individual type it is within the species, eg a lemon thyme will have the same therapeutic properties as a common thyme, etc.[5]

Tea and Sugar's Role in Kombucha

Tea (*camillia sinesis*) is very nutritious (especially in its unfermented green form, *see* p.52). It is high in fluorides and has anti-carcinogenic properties; it provides nitrogen, minerals, vitamins, and other substances essential for nutrition, and promotes the growth of the micro-organisms and the cellular construction of the Kombucha culture. Green tea is also high in vitamin C.

Sugar plays an essential part in Kombucha's brewing process, providing a nutrient solution for the culture, assisting in the feeding and respiration of the micro-organisms, and activating the yeasts. It also gets the fermentation process going. The yeast cells make certain organic acids, vitamins and supplementary yeasts, while the bacteria produce carbonation, ethanol and other organic acids. The bacteria break down the sugars into acetic acid and carbon dioxide.

The Importance of Polysaccharides in Cancer and Digestive Disorders

Sugars also play a part as polysaccharides, which form the fundamental connective tissue of all human organs. Their ability to cope with metabolic waste products is a crucial part of a healthy body. The Japanese have conducted interesting research with these substances within the area of immunotherapeutics, very much the domain of Kombucha therapy. These tests focus on the role of polysaccharides which are found in Kombucha and their positive effect on macrophages and T-cells. One trial showed that the survival rate in cancer sufferers given polysaccharides was twice that of patients undergoing conventional treatment. A German naturopathic clinic in Gaggenau, Germany, did trials which showed the curative effects of polysaccharides on gastrointestinal ailments as well as cancers.[6]

Symbiosis - Working Together and Restoring Balance in the Body

The German microbiologist and cancer researcher[7] Prof. Gunther Enderlein (1872-1968), developed the theory of pleomorphism (many-formedness) which is now becoming established worldwide. This is based on the idea that microbiological life goes through cycles from very primitive forms of virus through bacteria to fungi. They exist in all these forms throughout the human body, their balance depending on environmental factors both inside and outside the body. When they are 'symbiotic' or mutually dependent, there is health, and when in disharmony disease is likely to result. Enderlein was particularly interested in how groups of microbes interacted with one another.[8]

Just as Nature requires a balanced diversity of life forms in the natural environment, so it does in the microbial ecology of our bodies. So, as long as we don't ingest manufactured chemicals and pollutants or expose our bodies to stressful conditions which might disturb this diversity, there will be a healthful balance in the microbial life. Few of us are able to live a purist lifestyle, no matter how aware we are of the negative effects in this modern world. This is why we need to take a course of action, like Kombucha therapy, that detoxifies our system, in order to keep our internal microbial ecology healthy.

The Question of Candida

The opposite of symbiosis is dysbiosis, working against each other as in disease. Enderlein was the earliest contributor to a better under-standing of the vexed question concerning Candida, a yeast fungus in our bodies that has since got out of hand through the widespread use of antibiotics. [While antibiotics are used to destroy the pathogenic (harmful) bacteria in the body, they also destroy, or severely damage, the friendly bacteria as well.] It is now widely recognised that the common fungus Candida is found in two forms; one that can live symbiotically with the body microflora and which is *beneficial*, and the other better- known pathological form, which is often the result of a self-defensive mutation caused by antibiotics, and is *harmful*.[9] The latter is usually treated by an anti-fungal antibiotic with limited effectiveness, because its action is usually short-lived, allowing the pathogenic form to return. Candida is thought by many naturopaths to be one of the most invasive forms of fungal pathogens, responsible for, or contributing largely to, many serious illnesses today, including Multiple Sclerosis, Chronic Fatigue Syndrome (ME - myalgic encephalomyelitis) and cancer.[10] The gut is usually the primary site of pathogenic candida, and we have many reports from candida sufferers that Kombucha tea has helped to control it. (*See* Candida, page 78)

A typical yeast in Kombucha, saccharomycodes, does not have spores and is not in the candida family. It is therefore antagonistic to the troublesome yeast that infects so many people. Whereas most ascomycetes such as those found in penicillin, ergot, bread mould, mildew, thrush and others reproduce by means of spores, most yeasts reproduce vegetatively by budding. The Fission yeasts reproduce by means of fission-like bacteria, they don't bud or have spores. The pombe fission yeast of the Kombucha culture belongs to this type and is beneficial to Candia sufferers.

Adaptogens - Balancing the Body

Another feature of Kombucha is that, biochemically speaking, it is an adaptogen, that is a substance which has no harmful effects, but which works on a wide variety of conditions by 'normalising' the metabolism of the body, and bringing it back into balance.[11] So, for example, if you have high blood pressure, an adaptogen substance will lower it, and if you have low blood pressure, it will raise it. Kombucha's adaptogen effect is seen mostly through its effect on the liver, the blood and the digestive system, where it normalises the acidity or pH.

The Acidity Factor

The acid-alkaline balance is vital to human metabolism. It is measured by the pH (potassium/hydrogen) scale which goes from 0-14. The lower numbers are more acidic, the higher ones more alkaline. The pH of our body's cells is constantly responding to the food that we eat, the air that we breathe, and to our emotional state. The body has a remarkable balancing system that maintains the different organs at the pH level each requires for health. A pH of 7 is that of water, neither acid (lower number) nor alkaline (higher number).

The pH of your urine and saliva are indicators of the health of your digestive system: 6-7 for urine and 7-8 for saliva; the stomach is normally much more acid, at 1-2; the pancreas is happy at 7-8, and the large intestine at 6·5-6·9. The blood's acidiy is the most critical, and variation outside the normal 7·36 -7·44 can be serious. A cell's pH level is affected by toxins, which create more acidity. The body gets rid of toxic acids by various means. One is through breathing - that is why deep breathing is so therapeutic - it makes the blood more alkaline. Another is by flushing out - one of Kombucha's roles is to flush out the toxic acids through the kidneys.

We have seen how lactic acid helps balance the acidity of the gut. We believe that Enderlein's discovery that the blood has a vital microbiological life indicates how Kombucha can balance the acidity of two of the other vital organs of the body, the liver and the blood.

The Liver Filters Toxins

The liver is vital to life; it has the ability to restore itself and has many functions - to assist digestion, to store important vitamins and minerals, to metabolise proteins, fats and carbohydrates to provide energy for the body, to recycle red blood cells, and remove toxins from the body. Because of its role in pH regulation and of its detoxifying acids, Kombucha is a valuable restorative of liver function.

Blood - Brings Life to the whole Body

The blood is composed of red, white and T-cells, and plasma, that circulates, carrying nutrients, oxygen, waste products and many other substances around the body. Some have compared its purpose to that of living water in the earth, without which life would not be possible. Blood is like a separate organ, and has a health and balance of its own that is independent of the liver. When blood gets too alkaline calcium tends to crystallize out of the blood solution.[12] These crystals are deposited near the joints, causing joint tenderness, arthritis, rheumatism and allergies. Older people's blood becomes more alkaline, which can affect their circulation, oxygenation and energy. An acidic blood condition can lead to diabetes where fat and protein wastes are not being discharged. Another acidic condition results i7n adrenal depletion and general exhaustion. Any therapy that can assist the blood to keep its pH balance under adverse conditions is really valuable; and that is the effect of Kombucha.

Conventionally, blood is thought to be sterile. But through his dark-field microscope research, Professor Günther Enderlein has shown that it is teeming with microbiological life. Normally these micro-organisms are in a mutually beneficial state of balance (symbiosis) but, for example, the lowering of the oxygen content of the blood, nutritional deficiency and toxicity may lead to the development of pathogenic microbial flora which can result in disease in other organs of the body. These micro-organisms can apparently travel freely between the blood plasma which surrounds the blood cells, and the interstitial fluid which surrounds the fixed tissue cells of the body.[13] This discovery has important implications for Kombucha therapy, because Kombucha is known to have a balancing effect of the pH of the blood which is likely to make it less hospitable to pathogenic bacteria. This is clearly an area of much needed further research.

Energising and Balancing

Many people report a sensation of "feeling energy coursing through their veins" on their first taste of Kombucha; this response needs to be tested by observations in the laboratory. Many people with high blood pressure taking Kombucha have reported a long-term reduction in their blood pressure. Because our blood and its related fluids are all-pervasive with every cell of our bodies, the feeling of energy boost that is commonly reported by many Kombucha drinkers must be related to a beneficial action in the blood.

Of the various actions that Kombucha seems to manifest, we feel that the balancing effect will turn out to be one of its most important - as we shall see in later chapters (eg Chapter 12).

Kombucha is Not a Cure-All

During times of stress or ongoing imbalances in lifestyle and nutrition, the body and organs are weakened and gradually underperform. A disease or illness will eventually manifest, giving rise to a whole host of conditions - arthritis, poor eyesight, skin disorders, oedema, asthma, Chronic Fatigue Syndrome, or just poor energy. The list is endless, because each person has his or her weak area in the body. When the functioning of the body is improved and strengthened with Kombucha therapy, a symbiosis or balance is regained and a person's individual symptoms can consequently be relieved.

Kombucha is not a cure-all or a universal panacea of all ills, because many other factors which affect good health need to be taken into consideration, such as diet, exercise, lifestyle, emotional outlook and psychological make-up (depression, anger, grief, etc.), as well as the length of time a person has had a particular imbalance or disease.

When we are feeling low with a prolonged illness or just very tired it is very hard to take positive steps towards a better lifestyle and health. Kombucha therapy plays an important part in assisting the body to function properly, by helping to relieve some symptoms and giving us the energy and encouragement to continue to improve our health. It is empowering. This enables us to take a long look at ourselves to see where we may have created our own imbalances and what other positive changes we can make to create a better environment in which to function and improve all areas in our lives. (*See* Chapter 11)

Kombucha tea is not only taken by people with disorders or illnesses, it is also used as a preventative therapy to keep the body functioning well.

To Summarize

Although Kombucha's effects are individual, the most commonly observed are:[14]
- balancing the metabolism
- cleansing the blood and regulating the acid/alkaline levels in the body
- improving liver, gall bladder and digestive function
- detoxifying the body and enhancing the immune system
- raising energy levels

Extravagant Claims: Will Kombucha Cure Anything?

There are many apocryphal stories about how Kombucha will cure anything. Various books make such claims, and the Internet contains some extravagant assertions on its Kombucha pages, quoting numerous 'facts', some of which are mutually contradictory. This confusion, as we see it, is caused, or at least made worse by the modern shortcoming of studying subjects in isolation, and also by contemporary commercial hype which insists that we must expect certainties of cause and effect - i.e. 'this product will produce that benefit'.

Modern Medical Expertise

The modern medical 'expert' is one who has studied in great depth, for example, the action of a certain hormone on the liver, but who probably has a very unsophisticated idea of the causes and treatment of back pain, or the way in which the whole body is interconnected. The results of such a narrow view can be observed everywhere, with threatening health and environmental disasters looming around the world. The challenge facing science today is to embrace a truly holistic view of the way all life is interdependent, so that solutions which are Nature-friendly can be activated before it is too late.

Technocrats or experts in specific areas are highly valued in today's society. They may have little understanding of symbiosis (how people or other life forms coexist for mutual benefit). Nor do many of them seem to be aware of the intelligence and values of older societies whose people saw life as a broad canvas. These simpler communities understood about natural rhythms and the wisdom of encouraging the interdependence of and the inter-connectedness between all people and Nature.

Society's Folly

When you add to our culture's high level of expectation and need for immediate gratification, the powerful pressure from product promotion and advertising (much of it at an unconscious level as on television), can be a kind of brainwashing, and an inability to think for oneself. This can be extremely disempowering for the individual. But there are signs that people are beginning to think more for themselves and, ultimately, it will be people power that makes the changes. Membership of environmental organisations in the UK is now greater than that of all the political parties put together!

Why Don't all Doctors Prescribe Kombucha?

We are often asked "If Kombucha is so wonderful, why don't all doctors prescribe it, and why is it not more widely accepted?" This is largely a question about medical orthodoxies, political agendas and self-empowerment. (*See* Chapter 11).

The Western World is becoming Malnourished!

It is well recognised that a high percentage of the Western population is getting insufficient nourishment from modern diets and, as a consequence, our health, and that of society as a whole, is suffering. Kombucha is a food rich in vitamins and minerals which are essential to good health. Many doctors believe that supplementary vitamins and minerals are unnecessary, saying that we get sufficient of these in a balanced diet. While that may be true in theory, who gets a really balanced diet now? Much of the food that we purchase, even so-called 'fresh food', has been grown with chemicals - herbicides, pesticides and fertilisers. After this, they are sprayed with even more chemicals to preserve their colour and shelf life.

Many of the fast foods that we eat are processed to the point where most of the beneficial nutrients have disappeared altogether, leaving the meal virtually barren. The nitrogen fertilisers used in commercial agriculture stimulate plant growth too rapidly for the uptake of the trace elements and minerals essential for our bodies, resulting in the food lacking nutritional value. British government studies show that our intake of essential minerals and vitamins has fallen greatly since 1936, before the 'chemical revolution'.[15] The truth is that in the Western world we are malnourished![16].

As Hazel Courtney[17] tells:*"Over 50,000 chemicals are either being sprayed on fruits, vegetables and grains, or added to our food. Many of these chemicals have now entered the food chain and we are reaping a bitter harvest. Our fruits and vegetables contain substantially less vitamins and minerals than they did 50 years ago, sperm counts are dropping, overuse of antibiotics is causing new resistant strains of bacteria which trigger food poisoning. What is happening today, with the tidal wave of illnesses from heart disease, diabetes, candida and high blood pressure to asthma and arthritis, is that our bodies are telling us they have had enough. It is imperative that we wake up and educate ourselves and others in ways of protecting ourselves and our planet."*

Many people, including doctors and scientists, don't realise how much our immune systems are vulnerable to the effects of sophisticated forms of pollution. There are also the chemicals added to our food (both in farming and in food processing) that are supposed to make us enjoy them more. These are not friendly chemicals; they destroy the body's functioning, cause allergic reactions, digestive disorders and pollute our blood - they are poisoning us! In the worst cases, of the common prescribing of powerful drugs like antibiotics, cortisone and steroids, the homeostatic balance of the body is disrupted. As you will see in the case histories in Chapter 10, some people who were suffering from the side effects of these drugs believe that Kombucha therapy was in great measure responsible for restoring their metabolic balance and health.

Complementary Medicine

We do not wish to be critical of all doctors, many of whom have a real calling to heal, and most of whom are very supportive of and helpful to their patients. However, when we see the insights brought by the holistic view into the understanding of balance in the individual in relation to disease, we wish there was more cooperation between the traditional doctor and the alternative health practitioner. We both really believe in complementary medicine, where orthodox and alternative can each have its place and assist the other. Many doctors, afraid of being criticised by their peers, have privately supported their patients taking Kombucha tea. We hope that now they will become aware of the extensive research that has been done, especially in Germany and Russia, and will start to advocate Kombucha therapy more publicly, so that it can have a beneficial effect on a much wider population.

REFERENCES

1   Coined by Monica Bryant, BSc, Int'l Inst. of Symbiotic Studies, *Jour.Alt.Med.*, Feb.1986).

2   Bryant, Monica, "The Shift to Probiotics", *Jour.Alt.Med.*, Feb.1996)

3   Fasching, Rosina, *Tea Fungus Kombucha: The Natural Remedy and its Significance in cases of Cancer and other Metabolic Diseases,* Ennsthaler, 1991.

4   Frank, Günther, *Kombucha: Healthy Beverage and Natural Remedy from the Far East,* Ennsthaler, 1991.

5   Kusmirek, Jan, "Synergy - Close Encounters of the Plant Kind", *Aromatherapy Quart'ly,* 1994.

6   *Explore!,* vol.6, no.1, 1995.

7   Enderlein, Günther, *Bakterien - Cycologenie,* Semmelweis Inst., 1981.

8   Bryant, Monica, "Microbiology at a Turning Point", *Jour.Alt.Med.*, Mar. 1996.

9   Odds, *Candida and Candidiasis,* Ballière Tindall, 1995.

10 Chaitow, Leon, *Candida Albicans,* Thorsons, 1995.

11 Lark, Dr Susan, "Ginseng - the 'upper-fixer' of the biochemical world", *Health-Life,* Apr. 1995.

12 Pascal, Alana & Van der Kar, Lynne, *Kombucha: How-to and What It's all About,* Van de Kar Press, 1995.

13 Enby, Erik, "Mikrobliknande bildningar i blod vid kronsika sjukdomar" ("Microbe-like formations in the blood of patients with chronic diseases") *Swed.Jour.Biol.Med,* 1, 1984

14 Tietze, Harald, *Kombucha - The Essential Handbook,* Gateway, 1995.

15 a) "Mean Daily Intake of Vitamins", The Dietary and Nutrition Survey of British Adults, (Social Survey Div., Office of Population, Census & Survey, HMSO, 1990).

    b) Comparing the mineral values of a typical basket in 1936 (raw carrots, old potatoes, cauliflower, celery, chicken, beef, lamb, pork & cod) with 1987, there was on average, 68% more iron, 60% more calcium (calcium & iron deficiences are prevalent in young people today), 21% more potassium, 63% more magnesium, 34% more phosphorus in our food in 1936 (McCance,R.A. & Widdowson,E.M.: *The Composition of Foods:* Roy.Soc.of Chem. & MAAF, 1991).

16 The herbalist, Jill Davies, notes in her herbal home guide *Self-Heal* (Gateway, 1998) that, during his time as a hunter-gatherer (from pollen evidence), man collected and consumed between 100 and 200 different plant species. This diversity of chemistry would have protected his/her immune system and stimulated the digestion better than our modern diet. Modern man's normal dietary range is only between 20 and 40 species, whose chemistry is far from that of the original plants. Animals haven't fared any better.

17 Hazel Courtney is *The Sunday Times* health columnist, and author of *What's the Alternative?*

CHAPTER 4

SUMMARY OF KOMBUCHA RESEARCH

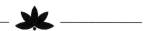

There is extensive literature dealing with the therapeutic effects of drinking Kombucha tea. The bibliographic references at the back of this book number over 200 and represent only a partial list. The total number of publications on Kombucha must now be nearly 300. So, if scientists insist, as several have claimed in media discussions we have had about our experience with Kombucha therapy - there is no scientific evidence that drinking Kombucha has health benefits - you have to ask what is their agenda? Inevitably it transpires that they have not read any of the research on Kombucha, even when offered, and probably won't even bother to. This attitude to us is certainly not scientific. Many of the media's producers and presenters justify this curious policy as giving a 'balanced view'. More truthfully, it is a hallmark of our 'adversarial' culture.

The Communist Experiments

In the early 1950s, after discovering that those communities in the USSR who were drinking Kombucha in areas of heavy industrial pollution seemed to be protected from the toxic climate, the Central Biological Institute in Moscow carried out extensive microbiological tests. They found the samples of Kombucha they took from these communities contained glucuronic acid and lactic acid - both anti-toxins produced by a healthy liver; usnic acid (an antibiotic), folic acid, B vitamins 1, 2, 3, 6 and 12. They isolated the bacteria: *bacterium xylinum, bacterium xylinoides*, and *bacterium gluconicum*, and the yeasts: *saccharomyces ludwigii, saccharomyces apiculatus* (varieties), *saccaromycespombe, acetobacter ketogenum, torula* varieties, *pichia fermantans*. Günther Frank reports that it was this research from the 1950s which first noted that the local climate, the water and the varying geography of the area affects the type or species of yeasts and bacteria found in a particular culture sample. Although there was a wide variation in the microbiological composition of their samples of the Kombucha culture, this did not seem to affect the typical way in which the brew seemed to work in the human body (*See also* page 18).

The doctors involved in this research became casualties of Stalin's anti-Jewish pogrom, and it seems that this put a damper on further research being done in Russia at that time. Incidentally, President Ronald Reagan was one who benefited from the Russian experiences with Kombucha. His cancers were alleviated after a sample culture was procured for him from Japan and he began drinking the Kombucha tea.

A Hundred Years of Research

Most of the research on the benefits of Kombucha has been done by individuals rather than groups. Among early reports were those listing the benefits of Kombucha for stomach, digestive and intestinal disorders. The following is a note of some of the principal researchers, with a very brief summary of their findings:

1914: Bacinskaya noted its effectiveness for gastro-intestinal activity. She recommended a small glass of Kombucha to be drunk before every meal.

1915: Prof. S. Bazarewski, researching indigenous traditions, found that the Baltic Latvians had a folk remedy of a 'wonder mushroom' that, besides alleviating headaches, had "wonderful healing power for many diseases".

1916: Prof. Dr. Lakowitz discovered that the mushroom quickly removed many gastric illnesses and nervous headaches, as well as helping digestive disorders.

1917: Prof. B. Linder noted its use as a regulator of intestinal activity, and as a cure for haemorrhoids.

1918: Prof. Dr. R. Robert recounted an anecdote describing it as an "unfailing remedy against joint rheumatism".

1926: Prof. Dr. W. Hennenberg told how, while on a visit to Russia, he heard about 'tea-kvass', a drink made from a tea mushroom which was "a remedy against all sorts of disease, especially constipation".

1927: Dr. Madaus made the first association between the ability of Kombucha's metabolic products to regenerate cellular walls and its resulting value in helping arteriosclerosis.

1928: Br. M. Bing also recommended the remedy as very effective for arteriosclerosis, but also for intestinal deficiency and gout, kidney stones and brain artery calcification, high blood pressure, eczema, headaches, irritability and anxiety attacks.

1928: Prof. Br. Lokowitz confirmed the efficacy of Kombucha for digestive upsets, and added that headaches and nervous disorders could be alleviated.

1928: Dr. L. Mollenda reported that the remedy was very effective for digestive disorders and arteriosclerosis, and also good for rheumatism, gout, kidney stones and gallstones. In addition, he found that angina treatment was enhanced. He observed that, despite the acidity of the brew, it did not make the stomach more acidic.

1929: Dr. E. Arauner summarised a number of medical reports on Kombucha by saying it helped diabetes and all aging problems, such as arteriosclerosis, high blood pressure and its consequences - dizziness and gout. He noted that Asian people in his country used it for the foregoing, and also for tiredness and nervousness. He also claimed that not only had professors, doctors and biologists confirmed surprising healing with Kombucha, but those that drink it reported "entirely excellent effects on the general body functions".

1929: Dr. S. Hermann described experiments with cats that had been poisoned by an anti-rickets vitamin D preparation. He noted that Kombucha lowered their cholesterol level. He concluded that it should also help arteriosclerosis where there was also a raised cholesterol level.

1944: Dr. H. Irion, who ran a college for chemists in Braunschweig, documented Kombucha's remarkable ability to invigorate the body's entire glandular system and metabolism. He recommended its use for all aging problems and intestinal disorders. He noted also that it helped the removal of deposits of excess fat, of cholesterol and uric acid.

1954: G. F. Barbancik wrote one of the first books devoted to the therapeutic properties of Kombucha which he discovered through its use at the Omsker Hospital in Russia. He reported successful treatment of tonsillitis, inflammatory diseases, dysentery, high blood pressure and acid-deficiency of the stomach.

1959: I. N.Konovalow reported that the varieties of bacteria and yeasts found in the Kombucha culture suppressed the growth of other species of yeasts and bacteria.

1961: Dr. V. Koehler reported encouraging results in the treatment of cancer with glucuronic acid, one of the constituents of Kombucha. He also noted surprising success with the treatment of trees suffering from disease caused by acid rain, exposure to radioactive fallout, sulphur dioxide, nitrites and ozone. He believed that it showed how valuable a detoxifier it would also be for the human.

1964: Dr. R. Sklenar of Oberhessen recognised the detoxifying properties of glucuronic acid in Kombucha for removing waste matter such as cholesterol and toxic deposits. He developed a biological cancer therapy based on Kombucha, and it is his recipe which is still generally used today for the production of the commercially bottled brew. He became a champion for the remedy, which he found helped invigorate the entire glandular system and the metabolism. He successfully treated arthritis, constipation, obesity, arteriosclerosis, impotence, kidney stones, rheumatism, gout and, significantly cancer, especially in its early stages.

1987: Dr. V. Carstens, wife of a former German President, recom-mended Kombucha therapy as a cancer prevention because of its properties of detoxification and improvement of the metabolism.

Conclusions of the Traditional Research

What comes up most often in this summary is the balancing of the glandular system and the metabolism, together with Kombucha's properties of detoxification and regulation of digestive activity. Apart from these, there are certain benefits that seem to be well established for Kombucha: its anti-aging properties, cellular strengthening, pH balancing, lowering of blood pressure, and general toning. Clearly there are now other health-promoting claims for Kombucha which need further research.

The Holistic Approach to Research

We feel it would be a mistake to conduct research based solely on extractions of the complex chemical constituents of the Kombucha brew, such as glucuronic acid for detoxification. Nature has created over centuries of evolution, in a way we cannot begin to appreciate, far less understand, complex organisms which interact with each other to maintain a precarious balance and interdependence which we interfere with at our peril.

It is the whole Kombucha organsm that is effective, not its constituents in isolation. This principle is at the heart of herbal medicine and is the main reason for its effectiveness and so too with Kombucha.

More productive would be specific research following the work of Günther Enderlein[1] on isopathy and symbiosis, which we touched on in Chapter 3. Also to be considered are the Japanese and German trials being conducted in the area of immuno-therapeutics with polysaccharides, an important constituent of Kombucha.

Energy Medicine

We make the case for Kombucha also as an energy medicine, which requires a rather different approach from that of the usual laboratory techniques. What is needed is more research working with people who have imbalances, to learn how healing works, rather than conventional analyses of a particular extract or of its effects on a specific symptom. The initiatives taken by Bob Banham in trials with MS patients (*See* Chap. 10, p.113) are particularly interesting. Current scientific thinking is still sceptical about any process whose workings are not exactly explicable scientifically. It appears that many people in conventional research do not make it their main priority to facilitate or possibly even to understand the healing process.

Investigations by the F.D.A.

In 1992 the Food and Drug Adminsistration which monitors food safety in the USA could find no fault with Kombucha tea. Their main concern was that it might become contaminated with the potentially harmful mould aspergillus. All the facilities for producing the beverage that they inspected were found to be satifactorily sterile, but they remained concerned about the level of hygiene in home brewing conditions. Did they not know that Kombucha had been brewed safely for 2,000+ years in ordinary home conditions?

There have been cases where misinformation campaigns have been initiated by persons or organisations who wished to discredit Kombucha and tried to identify it as the cause of an isolated death. None of these claims has ever been substantiated. People die from many causes, not least from the effects of prescribed drugs, but this is hardly ever discussed. Kombucha has a successful 2,000 year history, used by millions of people, by hundreds of doctors, medical researchers and some hospitals, each testifying to its effectiveness.

REFERENCE

1   Enderlein, Günther, *Bekterien - Cycologenie,* Semmelweis Inst., 1981.

CHAPTER 5

HOW TO BREW KOMBUCHA TEA SUCCESSFULLY

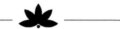

PREPARATION

In this section we want you to understand that brewing Kombucha is very simple, but we also want you to prepare yourself properly and to make a success of it straight away. Once you get the feel of how it is done, you will enjoy brewing Kombucha tea with confidence. So sit back and enjoy this chapter. Read it, read it again, and then begin.

Cleanliness and the Environment

Kombucha brewing is an adventure into the realms of microbiology which requires good standards of cleanliness. It is not necessary to use laboratory sterilisation procedures. Good, sensible kitchen hygiene is all that is required. It is essential to keep everything clean - your hands, what you are wearing, your surroundings and the equipment you use - both in preparing the brew and in its fermentation. Kombucha contains acetic acid which is a natural antiseptic, but even this will not be able to cope with a hostile and unclean environment.

Contamination is easily recognisable and shows itself as a mould, just as it would on yogurt or bread. This is the main concern for Kombucha brewers and the most common causes of mould are: insufficient heat in the fermentation process or placing the brew somewhere totally unsuitable like a cold, dusty broom cupboard or in a room full of plants where spores are in plenty!

These guidelines will help ensure a healthy Kombucha tea:
- Wash your hands with soap and hot water, and dry them on a fresh clean towel, or preferably use paper towels. Do not use a kitchen towel that has already been in use, as it will have bacteria on it.
- Ensure that all the equipment you use for brewing Kombucha tea is clean - you may prefer to keep it separate for this purpose. If you use kitchen scales, remember that flour is a major source of micro-organisms, so wash thoroughly to remove all trace.
- Keep the culture in a container covered in Kombucha tea or cold sweet tea until you are ready to use. Don't leave it to dry out on a plate for any length of time.
- The fermenting container needs to be in a warm, clean, dry and friendly environment where it will be undisturbed. The ferment needs to have some air circulating, so if you keep the container in an airing cupboard or hot linen closet, leave the door slightly ajar.
- The Kombucha ferment should not be kept near damp walls; spores are invisible to the naked eye and can easily be transferred to the Kombucha liquid.

Attitude

The reason you have decided to make Kombucha tea is because you care about yourself, your health and wellbeing. No one is going to do this better than you. No doctor or health practitioner, however good, can help you as much as you can help yourself.

Food grown and prepared with love tastes much better and does you more good than any industrially grown, processed or fast food you can buy. In the East, brewing Kombucha tea is traditionally regarded as a sacred ritual. A quiet time is chosen when every thought and care can be put into its preparation in order to make the best possible health drink for all the family. May we suggest to you that Kombucha's preparation continues in this tradition in the West, that you too consciously prepare your health beverage in the best possible frame of mind, with love and care.

You may find this example interesting: A friend of ours, Michael, an experienced dowser, was giving a workshop in which the energy fields of different liquids were being measured. The group dowsed two glasses of water, each from a different source which was not revealed to them. One was ordinary tap water and the other was water drawn from the springs in Glastonbury, England (which is regarded as 'holy' or healing water). The Glastonbury water dowsed as having a much bigger energy field (aura) than the tap water which had virtually none. However, after a pause Michael said, "Hold on a minute, try again". To everyone's amazement the ordinary tap water now dowsed stronger, and had a much bigger and vibrant energy field compared to the Glastonbury water. The difference was that he had blessed it!

We now pay much more attention to the way we prepare all our food and drink, including Kombucha tea. It takes time to change old ways, but we know that bringing the special and sacred into our daily lives makes a real difference, and affects the energies that we take into our bodies.

Keeping the Tradition Alive and Well

In Eastern countries, Kombucha was traditionally handed down from one generation to the next, family to family and friend to friend, each wanting to pass on the experience of improved health. In some Western countries it is becoming easier to find Kombucha, due to the recent upsurge in its popularity. In the UK, media interest shown in newspapers, magazines, radio and television, has helped enormously by reporting on the health benefits of Kombucha, and giving out the address of the Kombucha Tea Network UK. As a result, from a mass of enquiries, the dedicated coordinators of the Network have passed on thousands of cultures to new Kombucha brewers. Consequently, more and more people have been forming their own networks, and passing on cultures to their friends, families and neighbours. The vision that we had in 1993 is now becoming a reality. Soon it will be quite natural to know someone who can offer you a Kombucha culture and maybe, when visiting relatives or friends, will be greeted with an energising glass of Kombucha tea too.

Obtaining a Healthy Culture; Getting the Right Information

(Beware of Chinese Whispers!)

Many people, in their enthusiasm to give away cultures, either pass on a photocopied sheet of Kombucha brewing instructions that they had been given, make one up themselves or just give verbal instructions. These methods are open to corruption and we know that, as in the game of Chinese Whispers, by the time the message gets further on down the line, it has often changed beyond all recognition! I have been told by different people that they have been instructed to do exactly the opposite of what should be done. For example, a woman wrote to the Kombucha Network asking if it was correct to put her fermentation jar in the sunlight and to pass on only the thinnest 'offspring' cultures, throwing away the thicker ones! This is exactly what Kombucha doesn't like. It doesn't thrive in sunlight and the fact that she was producing thin cultures was proof that her brewing methods weren't working correctly. The reason she contacted us was that she was only able to make a drink that remained sweet and flat, even after 14 days of fermentation, and she hadn't noticed any real improvements in her health at all. Her instructions had been passed on by word of mouth from a friend who had obtained them in a similar way.

We explain to people the importance of getting the best available information on Kombucha; from a good book or from individuals who know what they are talking about. You need a top quality starter fungus in order to make the best possible Kombucha health beverage which will serve you and many generations to come. If you have been offered a Kombucha fungus from a friend, here are some guidelines that will help you to decide whether to accept it or to look elsewhere for a better one.

HOW OLD IS IT?
Ideally it is best to use a new fresh 'offspring' from a 'mother' fungus.

WHAT COLOUR SHOULD IT BE?
The type of tea used affects the colour of the Kombucha tea. If the giver used ordinary black tea, the Kombucha 'offspring' will be beige/brown, whereas if green tea was used, the 'offspring' will be a paler, whiter colour. Either is fine to use.

IS IT HEALTHY?
With clean hands examine the consistency and thickness of the fungus you have been given. It should look and feel quite rubbery and be difficult to tear. If it comes apart easily in your hands when pulled, discard it, as it has not come from a healthy brew. It should be of a reasonable thickness, approximately 2-mm/ $\frac{1}{16}$ th"- 4-mm/ $\frac{1}{8}$ th" or thicker.

Don't, on any account, accept a paper-thin offering, as this means that the brewing conditions or ingredients used by the previous owner weren't ideal.

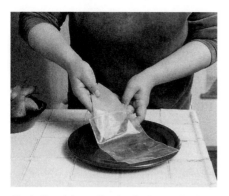

Fig.1: Receiving a Kombucha 'starter' culture through the mail.

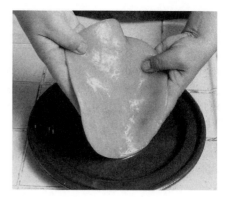

Fig.2: A healthy Kombucha culture

WHAT SIZE SHOULD IT BE?

It doesn't matter what shape or size the fungus is; all that matters is that it is healthy. A piece measuring at least 3-inches - whether square, oblong, circular, triangular or no particular shape at all - will work as well as a piece the full size of your batch brewing container. It doesn't even matter if it has got a hole in it or has a ragged edge; given the right ingredients and warm conditions a new fungus ('offspring') will form on top of the brewing liquid. That's the magic of Kombucha!

WHAT KIND OF TEA WAS USED?

Ordinary black (fermented) tea - Ceylon, Liptons, Typhoo etc, or green (unfermented) tea - Chinese or Japanese, or a combination of the two, have been proved to be the best for use in brewing Kombucha tea for optimum health benefits and for the continuing health and propagation of the culture itself. Some other herbs (and tea is a herb), such as nettle, dandelion and elderflower may also have been used for their healing properties in Kombucha. If so, it is better that they should have been used *in addition* rather than instead of tea.

NB: Some people mistakenly use fruit tea-bags wrongly marketed in supermarkets sometimes as 'herb teas'. These often contain only dried fruits and are not suitable for brewing Kombucha tea used on their own, as the health of the fungus would greatly suffer as a consequence. They can only be used *in addition* to tea. *(See* WHICH TEA TO USE - GREEN OR BLACK, AND THE QUESTION OF HERBS? page 52)

WHAT KIND OF WATER WAS USED?

Kombucha tea should ideally be made with chemical-free water (not straight tap water). Check that your supplier has been using filtered or boiled tap water, otherwise the culture's health and strength will be compromised. *(See* "Water - Why Chemical Free?", page 56)

WHAT KIND OF CONTAINER WAS USED IN THE FERMENTATION?

Make sure that the person who gives you your Kombucha culture has been brewing in a recommended container - that is, one made out of glass (Pyrex is good), china, high glaze porcelain or enamel (unchipped). All the experts agree that the healthful organic acids in Kombucha leach toxins and chemicals from containers made out of plastic (even food grade), aluminium, lead crystal glass, certain kinds of coloured glass and ceramic (where metals such as lead have been used in the glaze). It is important that you don't begin brewing Kombucha from an already toxic culture. (*See* "Which Container To Use?", page 38)

HOW WAS THE CULTURE STORED?

Ideally, your new Kombucha culture should be passed on to you immediately after it has been removed from the 'mother culture', and your fermentation should begin straight away. Most of the time, however, this just isn't possible, and cultures can be successfully stored for several weeks or months while waiting for a new home. A stored culture needs air to breathe and should be kept in the refrigerator, with a sufficient mixture of Kombucha tea and/or sweet tea to cover it, in a container made of glass or china etc.(not plastic) with a loose-fitting (ie. not airtight) lid. If your culture arrives in a zip-lock bag used for transportation, remove immediately and place it in a suitable container with some cold sweet tea and use as soon as possible. (*See* "Storing and Preserving Kombucha", page 67)

To obtain a Kombucha culture and for information and books (*See* "Resource Section and Suppliers")

Now you can begin your Kombucha tea brewing with confidence.

KOMBUCHA TEA - THE BATCH BREWING METHOD

SUMMARY OF EQUIPMENT AND INGREDIENTS (*See below for Recipe*)
Most of you will already have the equipment required for Kombucha brewing in the kitchen, so there probably won't be any need to spend money on a big initial outlay. Here's what you will need:

- a healthy Kombucha culture*
- a kettle or stainless-steel pan
- a 2½-litres/5-pints bowl made of glass, china or glazed ceramic that will hold 2-litres/4-pints of sweet tea and the 'starter' liquid, while leaving enough space above for the container to be carried without spillage.
- filtered tap water, or tap water boiled for at least 5 minutes
- tea - black, green*, or a combination of both
- white cane or granulated sugar
- scales or measuring cups
- a piece of muslin or thin permeable cotton to cover the bowl
- elastic to secure the cover
- a nylon sieve
- a funnel
- warm environment - airing cupboard, hot linen closet, clean boiler room, or use an electric heating tray* specially made for brewing purposes
- pH test strips* (indicator papers) for measuring the acidity level (optional)

- a simple thermometer*, for measuring the temperature of your fermenting Kombucha tea (also optional, but very useful)
  - * *See* "Resource Section and Suppliers"

The Recipe

This is enough for one person drinking the full recommended amount of 150-mls/1 wineglassful three times per day for 5 days.

INGREDIENTS:

A) USA
- 1 healthy Kombucha 'starter' culture
- 10-cups (5-US pints) of water
- 2-4 teaspoons (or tea bags) tea - black, green or a mixture
- ³/₄-cup white cane or granulated sugar*
- 2 tablespoons cider or wine vinegar - as a 'starter' (this is only used with the first batch if no 'mother tea'** is available. In subsequent batches use 1-cup/ ¹/₃-pint of the Kombucha 'mother tea' as a 'starter' and *omit* the vinegar).

B) METRIC - IMPERIAL
- 1 healthy Kombucha 'starter' culture
- 2-litres/4-pints of water
- 2-4 teaspoons (or tea bags) tea - black, green or a mixture
- 160-grams/5¹/₂-ozs (³/₄-cup) white cane or granulated sugar*
- 2 tablespoons cider or wine vinegar - as a 'starter' (this is only used with the first batch if no 'mother tea'** is available. In subsequent batches use 200-mls/ ¹/₃rd-pint (1-cup) of the Kombucha 'mother tea' as a 'starter' and *omit* the vinegar).

  * Do not reduce the amount of sugar or substitute brown sugar as this can prejudice the health of your Kombucha drink and life of the culture. (*See* "Why White Sugar, and can Honey or other Sugars be used?", page 54)

  ** The 'mother tea' is the fully fermented Kombucha tea used as a 'starter' for a new fermentation process (just as you would do in making yogurt).

Method

(For more detailed explanations see Chapter 6, "Kombucha - Your Questions Answered")
- Put loose tea or teabags into a teapot and pour the boiling water over (*Figs.3&4*), or with a pan - add cold water, bring to the boil and then add the tea.
- Allow to cool slightly, and add the sugar (*Fig.5*), stirring until it is dissolved. *Important - Do not add the sugar to boiling water.*
- Leave to brew for 10-15 minutes.
- Strain, if loose tea is used, otherwise remove the tea bags (*Figs.6&7*). Pour into the bowl or suitable container.
- Allow the liquid to cool to room (or blood) temperature and add the vinegar or 'mother tea' 'starter' (*Fig.8*).

- Now add the Kombucha culture (*Figs.9&10*). ***Important - do not add the culture to hot liquid as this will kill it.*** The culture may sink or float, it doesn't matter. It may remain at the bottom of the container for the whole of the fermentation time, this is quite normal. Make sure that there is a space of at least an inch between your Kombucha brew and the top of the container.
- Cover with muslin or a fine cotton that allows air in and will keep out fruit flies and other pollutants. Secure with elastic (*Fig.11*).
- Make a note on your kitchen calendar which day you started your batch. It is also useful to note am or pm, especially if your fermenting temperature is high, as an extra half day may be critical to the fermentation time.
- Put your container in a dark or shaded warm place 23°-30°C (70°-86°F), or on an electric heating tray, where it will not be disturbed and where there is some air circulation (*Figs.12&13*).
- Leave to ferment for 5-10 days (or more), depending on the temperature. You will notice a membrane beginning to form after 2-3 days over the surface of the container - this is perfectly normal and shows that the fermentation process is working. Begin tasting the liquid after 4-5 days. It should taste neither sweet nor sour. If there is still a sweetness in the beverage, cover and leave for another day or more until it has all gone. If the brew tastes sour and vinegary you will know that you have left it a little too long, and will learn to stop the fermentation earlier next time.
- When you are satisfied that your Kombucha tea is ready, with clean hands carefully remove the original 'mother' culture and the newly-formed 'offspring' onto a plate.
- Strain the beverage through a nylon sieve into bottles and place them in a refrigerator, or store in a cool environment (*Figs.14&15*). The Kombucha tea is now ready for drinking. Some people prefer to leave it for 5 days or so to develop a rounder, more mature flavour before consuming.
- The new 'offspring' can now be separated easily from the 'mother' culture (*Fig.16*). If by chance the two have fused together, simply snip them apart with sterilised scissors.
- You can now start your next batch either by re-using your original 'mother' culture or with your new 'offspring', if it is strong and healthy. NB: A Kombucha culture can be used successfully 6-8 times. If your new 'offspring' is quite thin, (which can happen with the first 1-3 brews), re-use the original 'mother' culture on its own or put the 'mother' and the 'offspring' *together* in the new fermentation. It is always better to begin a new batch immediately, if possible.

You are now ready to start drinking Kombucha tea and to experience for yourself its wide-ranging health benefits for all the family (*Fig.17*). For fuller explanations about the brewing process, and answers to many commonly-asked questions about Kombucha, please turn to the next chapter. Cheers!

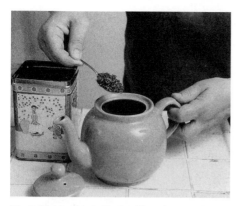

Fig.3: Making tea in the traditional way, using loose tea in a tea pot

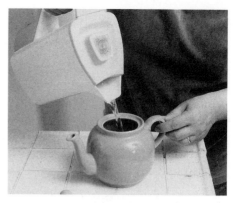

Fig.4: Pour boiling water onto the tea

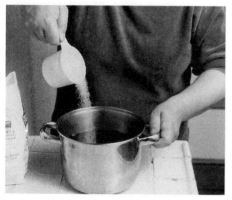

Fig.5: Cool slightly adding the sugar, stir to dissolve. Leave to brew 10-15 mins. (This picture shows using a stainless steel pan)

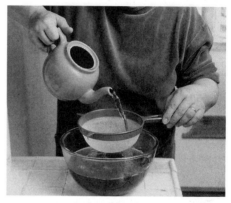

Fig.6: Strain tea into the bowl (or suitable container)

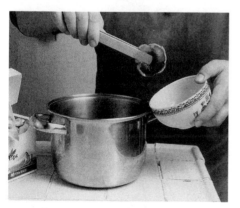

Fig.7: Otherwise remove tea bags from the tea pot or pan

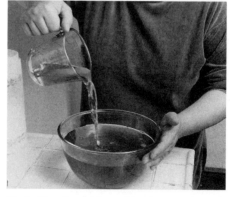

Fig.8: Allow to cool (room/blood temperature) and add vinegar or 'mother' tea

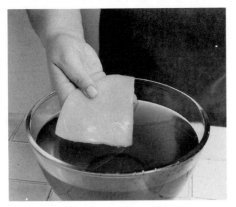

Fig.9: Add the 'starter' culture - a piece
8-10mm/3-4 ins. will work very well

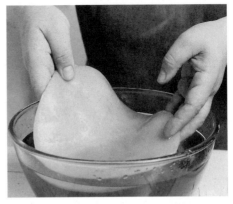

Fig.10: Using a large culture as a 'starter'

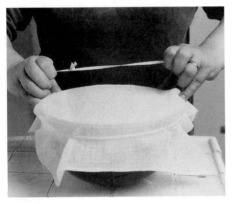

Fig.11: Cover with muslin or fine cotton and
secure with elastic

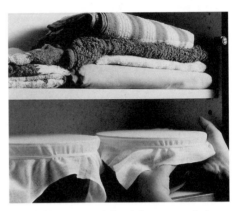

Fig.12: Put your container into a warm, dark
airing cupboard

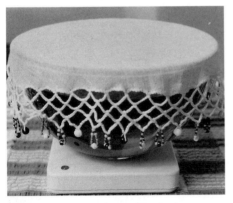

Fig.13: A bowl of fermenting Kombucha on a
small electric heating tray (useful if you don't
have a suitable warm place)

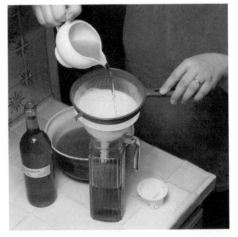

Fig. 14: Strain Kombucha when ready into glass
bottles or jugs.

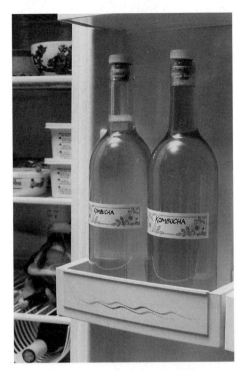

Fig.15: Refrigerate Kombucha or store in a cool environment

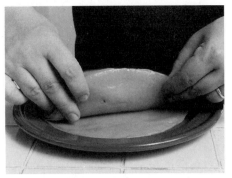

Fig.16: Separate the 'mother' culture from the 'offspring' to start another batch, or to give away to a friend

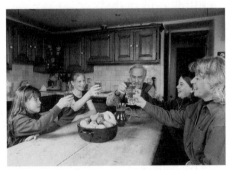

Fig.17: Good health for all the family

THE CONTINUOUS FERMENTATION METHOD
[Includes Making Larger Quantities]

This method of brewing Kombucha tea is ideal, especially if you are brewing Kombucha for a family and/or a number of friends:
- It is extremely fast and easy to make.
- You will always have sufficient Kombucha tea to give away, as well as having enough to put into that therapeutic bath.
- It is not so susceptible to variations in temperature as in smaller amounts with the Batch Brewing Method.
- The container which graces your kitchen, and its contents, becomes a good talking point with visitors who usually leave impressed and with a 'starter' culture of their own.

Many people from East European countries have told us they remember their grandmothers having a bowl of Kombucha on the shelf in the kitchen and just topping up as it was being consumed. This is a simpler method of Continuous Fermentation, and was a bit of a hit-and-miss approach to fermentation. Overall it will have done everyone the world of good, and we have ample written documentation to confirm this. We have been told that typically grandmother, who was so concerned for her family's health, would automatically dip a cup into the beverage as soon as you arrived to visit. It would depend on the particular stage of the Kombucha fermentation as to whether you were offered a sweet Kombucha tea drink (it wasn't quite ready) from a full pot, or a sour one (it had gone too far) from a half empty pot. We would imagine the days when the Kombucha tea was just right, neither sweet nor sour, were memorable days to visit Granny.

In the Continuous Fermentation Method of brewing Kombucha, as in the Batch Brewing Method, it is perfectly possible to achieve good results every time with a delicious drink that is neither sweet nor sour.

WHICH CONTAINER TO USE?

It can be any size, but typically anything from 12-pints upwards is suitable. We are very privileged to have bought one of the first traditional fermentation jars which are being made in the UK. They are thrown by hand from a high quality clay, have a non-lead glaze inside (very important) and are beautifully decorated on the outside. It has a wide neck opening which we cover and secure with muslin, and a hardwood tap several centimetres above the base for easy pouring, and to avoid draining the yeast sedimentation at the bottom of the liquid. They are available in two sizes, 16-pint and 26-pint. *(See Fig.19 and "Resource Section and Suppliers")*

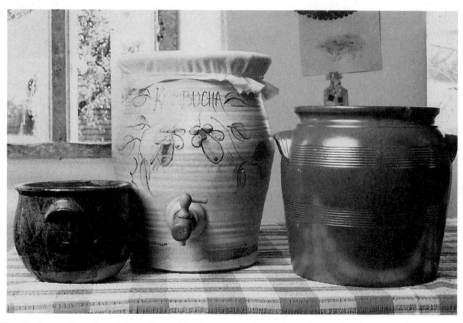

Fig.18: *A selection of containers for making larger quantities of Kombucha tea*

It is possible to use any large container without a tap *(see Fig.18)* like a bread crock or enamel container (without chips). You will have to scoop out your liquid from the top of the container with a ladle or jug which, although not quite so convenient, is no great hardship either.

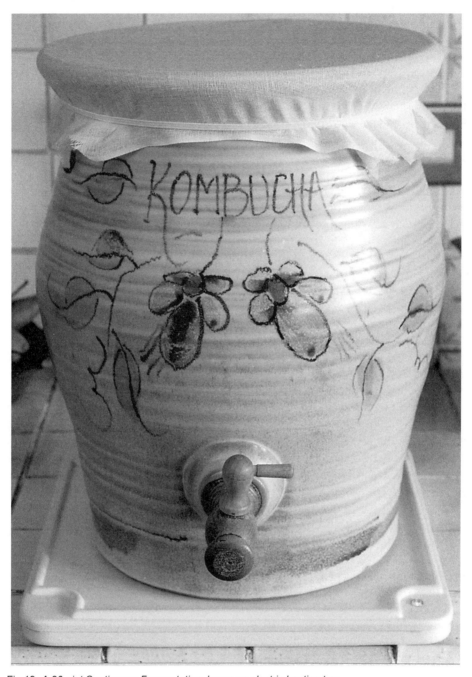

Fig.19: *A 26-pint Continuous Fermentation Jar on an electric heating tray*

The same guidelines apply to these larger containers as in the Batch Brewing Method, so *no aluminium or plastic*. Stainless steel is a good material to use as a container, they are easy to buy if not expensive. We have been asked many times if the barrels used in the home-brewing beer and wine world are suitable. They have a very small opening at the top, are usually made from plastic and are definitely *not* suitable for Kombucha tea, as it will leach toxins (even from food grade plastic).

FINDING WARMTH FOR THE FERMENT

A Continuous Fermentation container can be placed anywhere where it can be given the right warm conditions to ferment. However this large container, which needs a large volume of sweetened tea and will be very heavy, is dangerous if not impossible, to carry around. We find that the best and most convenient method when brewing in large quantities is to use an electric heating tray in a size made specifically for this method. It makes brewing large quantities of Kombucha tea safe and convenient to use (*See* "Resource Section and Suppliers").

THE 'STARTER'

When you are brewing larger volumes of Kombucha tea it is much better to use as much 'starter' Kombucha tea as possible - up to $\frac{2}{3}$rds of the full liquid volume. So for our 26-pint Continuous Fermentation Jar - we use only 24-pints (so that we can divide by 3) and would aim to use 16-pints ($\frac{2}{3}$rds) of 'mother tea' (Kombucha tea) as a 'starter'. A 12-pint container would aim to use 8-pints 'starter'. However, it is not always possible to have this amount of 'mother tea' 'starter' available, so you can use a minimum of 10% as in the Batch Brewing. (The reason $\frac{2}{3}$rds is advised will be revealed in the 'Method' below).

METHOD

• Work out the volume of liquid that your container can hold or that you want to make, and deduct from this the amount of 'starter' that you have available.
• Calculate the ingredients of tea, sugar and water in proportion to the Batch Brewing Method (*See* page 32) and make the sweetened tea. eg. - if you are making 6-litres/12-pints of Kombucha tea and you only have 2-litres/4-pints available as 'starter', you will need to make 4-litres/8-pints of sweetened tea, which is twice the recipe of the Batch Brewing Method.
• Allow to cool to room/blood temperature.
• Add the 'starter' and Kombucha culture (don't worry if it sinks to the bottom).
• Leave to ferment in a warm place or on an electric heating tray.
• When the Kombucha tea has fully fermented, ie. when it has lost all its sweetness, tap or take off only $\frac{1}{3}$rd of the whole volume of liquid and leave $\frac{2}{3}$rds behind as the 'starter'. *This is how you will proceed from now on.*
• Bottle and store in a cool place.
• **Important** - don't, as many people would naturally think, tap or take off one glass of Kombucha tea at a time just when you want to. When the Kombucha tea is ready, neither sweet nor sour, and is at optimum health benefits, you need to take the $\frac{1}{3}$rd volume off all at once. Drink only from this stored Kombucha tea, otherwise, if you keep on taking glassfuls beyond the point where your Kombucha tea is ready, it will have become more and more sour. It will also be difficult to calculate the amounts to replace.

• Top up with the same amount of sweetened tea - $\frac{1}{3}$rd, that you have just taken off and leave to ferment again. *It is as simple as that.*   Remember - don't top up with hot liquid!

Using up to $\frac{2}{3}$rds 'mother tea' as the 'starter' at the beginning is preferred where possible, as it enables the ferment to come to full strength straight away. If however, you only have 10% 'starter' Kombucha tea, it will probably take up to 2-3 ferments to reach its full strength and vitality. After that however, it will continue fermenting well and the Kombucha tea will have the full health benefits of all the organic acids, vitamins and minerals etc. By then it will also have the full bodied taste with the familiar 'zing' to it.

One might think that the whole brew would go more and more sour over the weeks and months of topping up, but it doesn't. However, try not to let a ferment go sour at any one time, as this will obviously have some effect on successive ferments, and will affect the taste of your Kombucha tea. You can top up with a variety of teas, made with the addition of herbs or dried fruit flavours. This makes Kombucha tea brewing an ever-changing variety of subtle flavours and interest.

HERE'S A TIP:
Instead of making the whole large volume of sweetened tea, make a smaller amount e.g. only boil $\frac{1}{4}$ of the volume of water needed. Add to this *all* the tea in a tea-pot or suitable container, cool slightly and then add *all* the sugar as well. Stir to dissolve and leave to brew for 10-15 minutes.

Now pour 150-mls/$\frac{1}{4}$-pint of the hot sweetened tea into a measuring jug and add 450-mls / $\frac{3}{4}$-pint of cold water. Then pour this into the Continuous Fermentation jar. Continue until you have made up the right amount of liquid which you want to use. This will bring it immediately to room/blood temperature, and you will avoid having to wait ages for a large volume of hot sweet tea to cool right down.   NB: This is only suitable if you are using filtered water and not when you have to boil it first, to disperse chlorine or to kill any bacteria.

HOW LONG WILL IT TAKE TO FERMENT?
Like the Batch Brewing Method, how long it will take to ferment will depend on the brewing temperature and the volume of liquid being made. In a warm cupboard it could take a large container anything from 7-10 days, whereas on an electric heating tray, it only takes between 4-6 days.

The Continuous Fermentation Method, which involves leaving $\frac{2}{3}$rds of Kombucha tea behind as the 'starter' and topping up with $\frac{1}{3}$rd sweetened tea, gives the ferment a strong beginning. With this higher proportion of 'starter' in its fermenting life, it therefore takes much less time for the full volume to ferment. Brewing Kombucha tea in large volumes is much easier than one would expect.

HOW BIG DOES THE KOMBUCHA 'STARTER' CULTURE HAVE TO BE?

It doesn't need to be as wide as the jar, but it is better to have a larger piece than you would have as your minimum of 8-10 cms/3-4 inches for the Batch Brewing Method. Although it is usual to be able to use a smaller piece of 'starter' culture than the size of your container, when you are brewing large quantities it is better to use a piece in proportion to the size of the container and the amount of Kombucha tea that you are making. A 'starter' culture too small will affect the overall strength of the ferment. A piece 15-cms/6-inches across or a whole circle of approx. 25-cms/9-inches from a batch brewing bowl would be ideal for a large quantity of approximately 6-12 litres/12-24 pints.

RE-USING THE CULTURE

There is no need to remove the culture from the fermentation jar until it begins to become invasive in the liquid or if you want to pass some on to a friend. New layers grow on top of the previous culture and fuse together each time you top up with a batch of the sweetened tea. As the layers build up, the underside ones slowly die off, so if you want to give a piece away take it from the *top* layer. We find it easier to take off the whole of the new culture that has formed every 2 weeks and we are then able to divide this lovely thick layer into portions to pass on to people. This prevents it building up too thick and having to slice off a top layer. You can re-use the 'mother' culture 6-8 times and replace it as necessary with one of the divided portions.

There is no need at any time to wash the culture under the tap, which will expose it to chemicals that are in the water. If you do want to remove the dark bits from underneath, which are dead cells, rinse it in some of the Kombucha tea with clean hands.

MAINTENANCE OF THE CONTINUOUS FERMENTATION JAR

Cleaning out the sediment that forms in the bottom of the jar is only necessary two or three times a year for a very large pot and more often with smaller containers. Your brew will tell you as you go along when it is necessary to do this. The first time we cleaned out our 13-litres/26-pint jar, was when we started to notice a cloudiness in the drink and a slightly yeasty taste after 3 months.

Remove the culture onto a dish and empty all of the Kombucha tea into bottles. Wash the container and yeast sediment out with hot water and allow it to drain. Start the whole process off again immediately - remembering to use $2/3$rds of the Kombucha tea as the 'starter'.

CHAPTER 6

KOMBUCHA - YOUR QUESTIONS ANSWERED

We know, from the many, many phone calls and letters that we have received over the last few years, and from those passed on to us by the Kombucha Tea Network coordinators, that Kombucha brewing raises lots of questions.

In this chapter, we take you through every step of making Kombucha tea in much greater detail, and giving fuller explanations to questions that you may have. The answers to other people's questions also often serve to illuminate new aspects of Kombucha therapy that you hadn't even thought of and we hope will serve to be interesting and informative .

If you don't find the answer to your particular problem here, do write to us with the details (*See* address for The Kombucha Tea Network UK, page 169). Not only will we try to help you but we will add any further information provided to later editions of this book so that others will benefit too.

GETTING STARTED

Q - How do I get hold of a starter fungus and how much will it cost me to start brewing?
A - The Kombucha Tea Network is the most reliable source in the UK if you want to be sure of getting a Kombucha fungus that has been grown in ideal conditions, with the greatest of care. (*See Fig.20 &* "Resource Section and Suppliers" for UK and other countries).

The Kombucha Network does not sell the Kombucha fungus, but charges realistic costs only. These have to take into account telephone bills, as there are often enquiries to respond to, brewing expenses, special packing materials and the price of posting your fungus to you. This is a labour of love,

but we have to be realistic. A small financial exchange should be made with a good heart. Many cultures are still given away free locally, to charities and people in need, both here and abroad. The Kombucha Tea Network UK also recommends using a good book, so that you have reliable information to refer to. Other countries will have their own arrangements and charges.

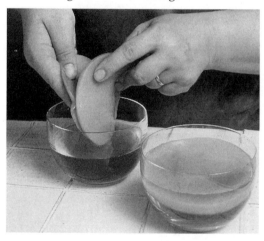

Fig.20: *Kombucha 'starter' cultures being prepared for the Kombucha Tea Network*

You will probably already have most of the basic equipment needed to get you started in your kitchen, including a suitable container which will hold 2½-litres/ 5-pints of liquid. Otherwise a 3-litre/ 6-pints - glass 'Pyrex' bowl can easily be obtained from hardware or kitchen stores. Thereafter, you will have to cover just the cost of your tea and sugar.

The other important consideration is to have sufficient heat for fermentation. Many people successfully use an airing cupboard or hot linen closet or some other similar warm situation in the home. (*See* "Heating Methods for Kombucha Tea Brewing", page 58)

Q - If I have acquired a starter fungus, but I'm not ready to begin brewing, what should I do?
A - Add 1 teaspoon of sugar to a cup of tea (without milk!) and allow to cool. Pour it over the culture, cover with a lid and refrigerate. Use within one week.

Q - Does it matter which way up the culture is when it goes into the sweetened tea, and what is the smooth side up?
A - At the beginning your culture will work equally well either way up, but after the first fermentation the under-side will gradually develop a dull brown film and it is important to keep this as the underside in further brews. The upper side, which remains the same colour and doesn't have the brown film, is the smooth side.

Q - What happens if my fungus sinks to the bottom of the bowl when I put it in, and it stays there?
A - It doesn't matter if it floats or sinks in the liquid. Given the right conditions and ingredients a new 'offspring' will always form on the surface of the liquid. You will find, probably within 2-3 brews when it is fully active, your 'mother' fungus will be more likely to float.

Q - I only have a sheet of instructions from a friend, is this enough?
A - Although making Kombucha is very easy, you will have questions as you progress and it is important to have the right information to hand. We have found that many information sheets contain incorrect information! Knowledge is vital when your health is at stake, so always obtain the best information that you can. If you have borrowed this book, go and buy your own copy, because the owner will probably need it back by now!

THE BREWING PROCESS

Q - What happens during fermentation?
A - The Kombucha beverage begins its life with a sweet taste which changes during the course of fermentation. The sweetness gradually disappears as the sugar converts into health-giving organic acids, vitamins, enzymes and minerals. Kombucha tea will give optimum health benefits when *all* the sugar has been converted.

It is important to know that one of these organic acids - acetic acid, which is the main component of vinegar, becomes more evident as the fermen-tation progresses. This accounts for the familiar slightly 'sour' taste that people often remark on with Kombucha tea. A sour vinegary taste is produced only when the fermentation has been allowed to continue too long. If the fermentation is stopped too early, however, the taste will still be sweet and the benefits will not be as great.

Your aim should be to produce a beverage that will both do you good and be enjoyable to drink. This will be just at the point when all the sweetness has gone. You will know you have achieved this **when the taste is neither sweet nor sour and the Kombucha tea has a 'zing' to it**.

Q - How long do I leave the Kombucha to ferment?
A - Much depends on the overall brewing temperature that you used as to how long your Kombucha is going to take to ferment. There is no set time, as it is very individual. A person with an airing cupboard or hot linen closet which is constantly warm, will brew their Kombucha in less time than say someone else's whose heating system is on low and is cooler overall, or that fluctuates going off for long periods at a time. Overall the brewing time will vary depending on temperature, heating method and volume of liquid used, but it will be between 5-12 days approximately.

Q - What should the Kombucha tea taste like?
A - Each person has their own idea as to when their Kombucha tea is ready, depending on personal taste. Try to stay 'in tune' with your fermenting Kombucha so that you learn to make it well and achieve the flavour you prefer. Do not be put off because you have so far only been able to produce a sour-tasting drink. When brewed correctly, Kombucha tea can be absolutely delicious. But to achieve this, you need to understand what is happening in the whole process, and how and what you are doing to affect the taste.

Some people enjoy and make their Kombucha taste like a sharp cider compared to others who achieve a more delicate, light Mosel wine flavour. We prefer the special combination of using Japanese green tea with dried elderflowers to produce a fresh, light taste, but with the familiar 'zing' to it at full fermentation time.

Though each batch is different, Kombucha usually has little bubbles of carbonic acid in it and is pleasantly effervescent. It is all a question of personal choice, but being better informed will enable you to make that choice rather than turning your Kombucha tea brewing into a hit-or-miss affair.

The taste and quality of Kombucha tea is affected in a number of ways:

- the type of tea used
- the addition of herbs, fruit, ginger etc.
- the quality and type of water used
- the health of the 'mother' culture
- the 'starter' Kombucha tea and its quality
- the temperature and method of fermentation
- the type and size of container used
- the length of fermentation time
- and of course the amount of TLC (tender loving care) that was put into it too

Kombucha tea making can become a fine art like wine-making, and people have been known to organise parties and have great fun tasting each other's and swapping tips. We even have a friend who decided to do something a bit different at her local church and organized a Kombucha tea party to bring interested people together for a tasting and information. Some parishioners had experienced great relief from their arthritic knees and the rest of the congregation wanted to know what the magic formula was! Kombucha is a great community builder.

Q - What should I do to test when the brew is ready?
A - A day or two before you think your beverage may be ready, remove the cover from your brewing container. You will see that a new 'offspring' culture, like a cream or whitish thick gelatinous skin, has begun to form *over the surface of the liquid* on top of your 'mother' culture . The new culture **never** forms underneath the 'mother' culture. Ease the 'mother' culture and 'offspring' aside and remove a little of the liquid to taste, with either a spoon or a small glass. If the Kombucha tea still tastes sweet, cover and leave it for another day or so and then re-taste. When the sweet taste has gone, then it is ready. If the beverage tastes too sharp or slightly vinegary, then it has been left too long, and you will make a note to taste and stop the fermentation sooner next time. (The Kombucha tea will still be all right to drink at this stage and you can always add some water or fruit juice if you want to make it more palatable.)

TESTING THE PH OF KOMBUCHA WITH TEST STRIPS (INDICATOR PAPERS)

Some people don't want to rely on just taste alone and want to be more exact in the way that they make their Kombucha tea. They would like to ensure that, when the beverage is ready, it is at the correct acidity level for optimum health benefits. This is especially important for diabetics and chronic fatigue sufferers. Accurate testing of the pH of Kombucha can be easily carried out using test strips (indicator papers). The test is simple:

Remove a small sample of beverage from the fermentation and dip a test strip paper into it. The colour of the paper will change and, after a few seconds, can be measured against a chart which will show if the tea has reached the correct pH or degree of acidity. The ideal pH value of fermented Kombucha beverage is between 2·6 - 3. If it hasn't reached an acidity reading in that range, the brew should be left another day or so and then re-tested.

NB. It is important not to dip the test strip paper directly into the fermenting beverage as the chemicals impregnating the paper would enter the brew.

(For pH test strips, *see* "Resource Section and Suppliers")

THE FERMENTATION TEMPERATURE
Q - What is the right brewing temperature?

A - Temperature is one of the most important factors to consider when brewing Kombucha tea. Using both historical research documents and our own experience, we have found that Kombucha ferments best at a temperature between 23°-30°C (74°-86°F). This is where the organic acids develop and a high level of concentration and antibiotically effective substances can be formed. Acetic acid bacteria develops best in the higher range and there is a good balance of bacteria and yeasts. In addition there will be a healthy and successful culture.

Although Kombucha can ferment reasonably successfully in a normal warm daytime room temperature it will have difficulties if this temperature falls significantly at night or fluctuates wildly during periods when the heating is off or the weather cools. Research shows that below 18°C (64°F) the activity of the bacteria is reduced, and only the yeasts work as they require less heat. There will also be more risk of contamination (mould). Many people have failed to make Kombucha tea successfully and given up because they didn't have sufficient heat. Others, fortunately, have contacted the Kombucha Network, with advice to increase the temperature for the fermentation and, hey presto, found that it worked! Of course, if you are lucky enough to live in a tropical country, your normal room temperature will be fine!

Q - Our hot water heating system goes off during the day while we are at work and comes on again in the evening so that there is a large fluctuation in temperature is this OK for our Kombucha ferment?
A - While the Kombucha brews more effectively within a constant temper-ature range, it will still be possible to make a Kombucha health beverage that will work well enough with some reasonable temperature variation. A large fluctuation however will be more difficult, as it will take longer for the fermenting beverage to come back up from the cold to the right brewing temperature where it begins to be active again.

Q - Why does Kombucha need to be in the dark?
A - Sunlight and ultra-violet light are harmful to certain micro-organisms and will inhibit Kombucha's vital processes. It is therefore important to keep your fermenting beverage and fungus in the dark or shade. If you have your container on a kitchen surface your Kombucha may be exposed to too much light. To shade it, fold a tea-cloth in half and place over the secured muslin cover, creating a small peep-hole at the front to allow air in. If you are using a glass container then place it inside a box or something suitable to shade the sides of the bowl as well.

THE DOSAGE

Q - How much Kombucha tea should I drink?
A - It is important for *everyone*, old and young, when starting to take Kombucha to begin with a **smaller** amount at the beginning and *gradually* to work up daily to the full recom-mended amount.

Take Kombucha three times a day *before* breakfast and *after* lunch and dinner/tea.

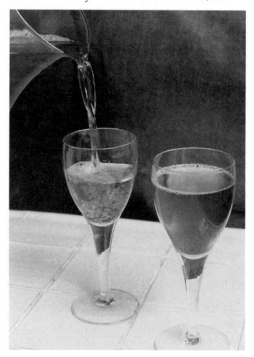

Fig.21: *A wineglass of 150-mls is the recommended amount to take three times a day*

Adults

The recommended full amount of Kombucha tea to take is: 150-mls/ one wine glassful three times per day. Start with 1-2 tablespoons, and gradually build this up daily until the full recommended amount is reached. (*See Fig.21*)

If there is an extreme weakness or illness, i.e. the elderly and people with ME (Chronic Fatigue Syndrome), MS and Cancer, begin with as little as 1 teaspoon and work this up daily to the recommended amount, or to what you personally feel comfortable with.

Children

Here are some guidelines for the recommended daily amount of Kombucha tea for older children with starting amounts in brackets. This can be reduced to as little as 1 teaspoon if there is extreme weakness or illness. (*See - "Contra-indications" below for infants and babies*)

- a child of 6-8 years 50-mls (1-2 teaspoons) three times a day

- a child of 8-10 years 75-mls (1 dessertspoon) three times a day

- a child of 10-14 years 100-mls (1 tablespoon) three times a day

Water, fruit juice or cordial may be added to make the drink more acceptable for a younger (or older) palate.

These amounts have been suggested through research and investigation and have proven to be ideal for the body to use for optimum benefits without overloading the system. There are times, however, when you might need some extra help such as in cases of cancer. The well-respected German specialist, Dr. Rudolph Sklenar, recommended that the daily amount could be increased (to about ½-litre) for the treatment of pre-cancer (the preliminary stage) and increased further in cases of established cancer to 1-litre per day (spread over a 24-hour period).

The above increases are to be regarded only as a recommendation for life-threatening illnesses and not as 'the norm'. In fact it can be harmful for those people in reasonable health to take too much Kombucha.

Some people, in their desire to get well, may be tempted to take the view about certain beneficial substances: "If a little does me good a lot will make me even better".

Even though Kombucha has been sensationalised over the years with names to tempt over-consumption, such as Miracle Cure, Tea of Long Life, Wonder Tea, Gift of Life, to name but a few, it is important to resist the urge to overindulge in Kombucha tea in the hope of feeling better faster. However good a food, drink or health supplement may be for you, you should never risk taking it to excess. In extreme - and, thankfully, rare - cases, carrot juice and even water have proved fatal when consumed in huge quantities. And the same applies to Kombucha. Overdosing on it could lead to your body becoming overloaded with the very substance that you took to do it good in the first place.

CONTRA-INDICATIONS

Q - Are there any circumstances when one should NOT drink Kombucha?
A - Pregnant women and nursing mothers are not advised to take Kombucha tea which will be too strong both for the sensitive digestion of a growing foetus or a young baby receiving it through its mother's milk. A parent or carer needs to follow their own instincts on the borderline of an infant and a child of 4 years old, by taking into consideration its health and strength. But always err on the side of safety by taking smaller amounts to begin with.

DETOXIFICATION

Kombucha has been proven in analysis to be a powerful detoxifier of the body and, in particular the liver and kidneys, mainly due to the effects of its glucuronic acid content. Detoxification symptoms are sometimes similar to those experienced in fasting and may include:

- headache

- stomach ache

- perspiration - which may smell stronger

than usual

- pimples
- an increased urge to urinate and/or defe-
cate - which may also be accompanied by
a stronger smell

These are all positive symptoms and simply
mean that your body is throwing off accumulated toxins that are overloading your
system, preventing it from working to its
maximum efficiency.

Being Kinder to Oneself

We advise *everyone* to ease in the detoxification process gently starting with a small
amount of Kombucha tea, then slowly and
gradually working up to the full recommended amount of three wineglassfuls a
day for an adult. In this way the symptoms
of detoxi-fication may be much lighter or
not even noticed at all. However, nearly
everyone notices that their bowel movements become more regular - which is no
bad thing. As a guiding rule, if you experience any discomfort at all, *stop* taking Kombucha for a day or two and then resume,
drinking a smaller amount and gradually
build this up at a rate which feels more com-
for-table to you.

Remember, the amount of Kombucha tea
that you start off with will vary depending
on your general health, the severity of any
illness, weakness or imbalance you may
have and also how your body reacts to it. It
is an ideal opportunity for you to begin
(sometimes for the first time) to really listen
to your own body and to take responsibility
for it by drinking Kombucha and consciously noticing how you are feeling while
taking it.

*Q - Can I take Kombucha continuously or do
I need to take an occasional break?*
A - It is wise, as with all kinds of medication
and supplements, to take a break from
Kombucha periodically. Otherwise the body
can become too dependent on it and may
begin to lose its effectiveness. We recommend that you leave off taking Kombucha
for a week at least every 2-3 months. Some
people decide to take one week off every
month or one month off in every six.

Choose whatever feels right for you - but
remember it is important to **take a break.**

One word of caution: If you are ill, or
there is an imbalance, you may experience a
return of your symptoms immediately after
you stop drinking Kombucha tea if you take
your first break too soon. If this happens,
resume taking Kombucha immediately and
leave your break until a later date when you
have begun to experience a more lasting
improvement. If you notice only a slight
setback when you stop taking Kombucha
tea, you will probably decide to continue
with the break, but make it shorter at the
beginning and build up on this over a period of time. So, be guided by your overall
health and stability, and use your intuition
and commonsense to decide how and when
to take your breaks.

*Q - Should I take Kombucha before or after
meals?*
A - Dr. Sklenar, a Kombucha pioneer from
Germany, suggests that the first glass
should be taken before breakfast on an
empty stomach and the rest during the day
after meals. The reasons are that he probably wanted to cover the broadest range of
effectiveness possible where Kombucha will
work on an empty or full stomach.

*Q - Should I continue to drink Kombucha if I
don't feel any benefit?*
A - It may be that you need to give Kombucha more time. After all, some of us have
given our bodies many years of gradual
abuse, through second-rate nutrition and
poor lifestyle, so it may take time before we
notice any real improvement and there is
always room for some more improvement!
Many people use natural medicine to prevent them from becoming ill.

*Q - Should I always drink the same amount
of Kombucha tea?*
A - You should go by how you feel and listen to your body. There is a recommended
amount, arrived at after much research,
which provides an effective guideline, but
some people feel better taking less than this.
There are no hard and fast rules as every
person is unique.

Q - Do you adjust the quantity of Kombucha beverage taken to the body-weight of an individual?

A - No, it depends on the person's health, and how toxic, well, weak or ill they are.

Q - Can animals take Kombucha?

A - Yes, but this time in amounts according to the size of the animal. A horse would have more, say, than a small terrier dog.

Q - What happens if I drink a jelly-like bit that has formed in the drink?

A - These small 'happenings' as we call them, that sometimes form in the 'live' beverage won't do you any harm, but you can avoid drinking them by using a fine mesh sieve (plastic is OK for this short time), every time you pour out a glass of Kombucha tea.

HEALTH QUESTIONS

Q - Why is Kombucha claimed to be a cure-all?

A - Articles in popular journals are frequently sensational and often claim this, but we certainly don't. What happens is simply explained - when the body is out of balance it complains and can thrown up a whole host of symptoms which manifest in different ways to different people. Each person has their own areas of weakness, e.g. the skin, stomach, liver, kidneys, joints etc. Kombucha sets to work cleansing, strengthening and balancing the body, helping it to work better and bringing it into a state of better health. In so doing, each person can experience their own individual symptoms subsiding or disappearing. This explains the long list of symptoms that Kombucha has supposedly 'cured' when they are in fact the ever-growing range of symptoms that many, many people have all been helped with.

Q - If it is so wonderful, why don't doctors recommend it?

A - We have found that those doctors who have read up on Kombucha or have used it with their patients generally encourage its use, such as Dr Campbell-Brown of the Kombucha Tea Network UK. Unfortunately some doctors may be concerned about disapproval by other doctors, and fearful of speaking openly about it. From the constant feedback we receive, we have learned of doctors who, on seeing improvements in chronic and stubborn conditions, have told their patients to continue taking Kombucha. Some doctors have even asked their patients for more information and a piece of culture so that they too can start brewing and drinking it themselves. We hope that this book will encourage and stimulate more interest among doctors.

Q - What is the scientific and medical evidence of Kombucha's effectiveness?

A - There is a great deal, mostly in German and Russian. Unfortunately most of it has not been translated into English. You can get the flavour of this research from the "Bibliography" at the end of this book.

Q - Why are some doctors so negative about Kombucha?

A - There are quite a few who are not. Those who are negative will not have bothered to read any of the documentation or research material available. They have learned to put their trust in synthetic drugs rather than natural products and seem to forget that these drugs originated in the natural world where they still grow all around us now, as Nature makes many plants available to us for our healing. Some doctors are sceptical of anything that has not come from a source given seal of approval by their own orthodox Western training. There is a growing number of doctors however who have open minds and whose main concern is for the whole health of the patient and wish to encourage self-empowerment.

Q - Is there danger from contamination in making Kombucha tea, this seems to be put forward as a potential risk?

A - Kombucha has a great capacity for regeneration. If it did not have this high biological energy, it would not have survived its long time span from the Chinese Empire more than 2,000 years ago. Warnings of it being dangerous to make Kombucha at home are mischievous and come from a perspective of ignorance, economic interest or a cynical medical profession. Follow the normal, sensible hygiene rules we suggest and you will come to no harm whatsoever.

Q - Are there any side-effects?
A - Yes - good health! Kombucha is a product of nature, and as such doesn't have the side-effects you might get with chemical drugs. The main effects to be aware of at the beginning may be those of detoxification, which may show as passing urine or faeces more frequently than usual, a headache or possibly pimples. These symptoms all pass and will leave the body cleansed and all the better for experiencing them. (Detoxification can be eased in more gently - *see* "THE DOSAGE", page 46)

Q - What happens if I have a reaction when I first start taking Kombucha?
A - Stop taking it for a day or two, then re-commence taking smaller amounts.

Q - Will Kombucha throw up a lot of symptoms together when I first start to drink it?
A - A few people have reported a 'healing crisis' when first using Kombucha. This can be scary if you don't know what's happening. The best way to avoid this is to drink only small amounts of Kombucha to start with and to gradually build it up.

Q - Can I become dependent on or addicted to Kombucha?
A - Not addicted, but it is always wise to give the body a break when using any kind of health supplements, so that it doesn't get used to them or they lose their effectiveness.

Q - Can I fast by drinking Kombucha tea?
A - You can use Kombucha only as part of a fasting programme, but don't drink more than the recommended amount, and take plenty of water also to assist the body in ridding itself of waste products and toxins.

Q - Will I lose weight with Kombucha?
A - Possibly, many people do. If Kombucha helps your body to metabolise, function and eliminate better, then you should lose weight.

Q - I have ME and Candida. I'm not supposed to have anything that contains sugar; does it matter with Kombucha?
A - You must make sure that all the sugar

has been converted in the fermentation process. Aim for a taste that is slightly on the acid side, indicating that the sugar has been completely converted, or use pH test strips to make absolutely sure.

Q - Kombucha is called a 'mushroom'; I am worried because I can't eat any fungi on a Candida diet.
A - Don't worry. Kombucha is known by many names, one of them the 'Manchurian Mushroom,' which is misleading because Kombucha is definitely not a species of mushroom.

Q - I am diabetic. Can I still drink Kombucha?
A - Yes, but it is very important if you are diabetic to use pH test strips or allow the taste to become positively more sour, which makes sure that all the sugar has been converted during fermentation. A close check should also be made on your blood sugar levels while drinking Kombucha and professional supervision would be wise to help monitor the situation. Do also check that you are able to take the small amount of alcohol of approx. 0·05% in Kombucha.

Q - What if I get diarrhoea?
A - It is not uncommon when you first start drinking Kombucha to be looser and more frequent in your bowel movements, because your system is having a clear out. If you get diarrhoea, you should reduce the amount you take for a while. It is also less likely to happen if you drink your glass of Kombucha Tea in small sips, instead of drinking a full glass all at once.

Q - Can someone with an acidic stomach drink Kombucha tea?
A - Kombucha is very good for digestive disorders when taken sensibly. Begin with a small amount, diluted, gradually building this up to the full recommended dosage. Also, don't allow the beverage to ferment until it is sour. Stop the fermentation immediately the sweetness has all gone.

Q - Are there some people who have a reaction to Kombucha and have to stop taking it?
A- One has to decide whether they are experiencing a detoxification and its symp-

toms, in which case they should ease back on the amount being drunk and gradually work through the detoxification process. To discover whether they are having a genuine

allergic reaction they could try a muscle test. (*See Fig.22*)

Q - How much alcohol is there in Kombucha tea - can alcoholics drink it?
A - The amount of alcohol in Kombucha tea is minuscule - approximately 0.05%, but this can vary slightly. Most recovering alcoholics are able to, and have benefited from taking Kombucha. However, there may be some who are sensitive even to the least amount of alcohol, and may have to avoid Kombucha tea as well. A muscle test would be worth trying to check if it OK to drink it. (*See Fig. 22*).

Q - How do I know if it's helping me?
A - Some people notice an improvement immediately. With others the effect is much more gradual. One day you may notice you are not getting that familiar headache or pain you usually get when under stress, or that your body is moving better and you are generally feeling more cheerful. Apart from Kombucha being a good insurance policy to protect your immune system, it is also a very important nutritional food, and will, over a period of time, make you feel stronger, brighter, more intelligent and energetic!

MUSCLE TESTING
This is a very simple technique that anyone can do at home if we have some uncertainty about a particular food or drink. We can then find out whether or not it is beneficial to us. A food which is good for one person is not necessarily good for another, and within a diet some foods are better for us than others and also at different times in our lives. Our bodies are constantly shifting and changing through our various ages, and the daily stresses and strains we put onto it. These can make us more susceptible to allergies or passions for certain foods. To maintain a balance in health we would be wise to eat or abstain from certain foods in

order to heal. It is very important to listen to our bodies needs, and muscle-testing is one way to help us do this.

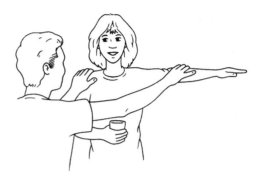

Fig. 22: Muscle Testing

HOW TO MUSCLE TEST KOMBUCHA
Based on the understanding and belief that the body has an intelligence and does not lie, you can communicate with it by asking questions with a 'Yes' and a 'No' answer.

The person being tested holds a sample of food or drink - in this case Kombucha tea, in their right hand close to the chest and extends their left arm out to the side. (*See Fig.22*) The tester places their left hand on the persons right shoulder and places their right hand onto the person's left wrist. A tension needs to be set up here where the person being tested resists pressure from the tester who is trying to push the arm down at the wrist - don't be too strong though, as a medium pressure and resistance is all that is needed.

The person being tested asks: "Is this Kombucha tea good for me?" If the answer is "Yes" meaning that it is beneficial, there will be a good resistance, but if the answer is "No", meaning that it is not beneficial, then the arm will weaken and give way to the pressure.

Before starting, try experimenting first with some obvious foods or substances that you know will be harmful to you, such as furniture polish or a bottle of turpentine. You only need a small sample of food e.g.; butter in a dish, a piece of fruit or use it whole, like an apple. With some fresh foods you may need to peel it first e.g. a banana - where the fruit inside may be beneficial to you but the skin will be harmful. So be precise with the food and questions you are asking, and you will receive the correct answer.

WHICH TEA TO USE - GREEN OR BLACK, AND THE QUESTION OF HERBS?

Q - What are black and green teas - and which is best to use?
A - Both come from the same tea bush, *Camellia sinesis*. Ordinary black tea of the kind commonly used in the West - such as Ceylon, Lipton's, English Breakfast, Typhoo etc - is *fermented*. Green tea (Japanese or Chinese) is *unfermented* and has many health-giving properties.

Black Tea - is often referred to in Eastern literature and was used for medicinal purposes. It was only later that it became a luxury, then a household item. Black tea is fermented before drying, which darkens the leaves and results in a brown-coloured beverage.

Green Tea - is not fermented, instead, as soon the leaves are picked, they are lightly steamed, during which oxidation occurs and the tannins and chlorophyll are preserved. Leaves are then rolled and dried. You can also buy semi-fermented teas such as Oolong (Formosa). In China and Japan, people are still known to eat the leaves after drinking green tea, because of their high mineral and vitamin C content.

Being British we enjoy a good quality cup of tea and have always thought that it made good sense to use a good quality tea for our Kombucha tea making. During the years we have been making Kombucha we have enjoyed a wide variety of flavours from using different teas. Black tea tends to produce a a stronger, fuller-bodied flavour, while green tea's taste tends to be lighter and fresher. We often mix them together.

Most historical scientific publications discuss the use only of black tea (compared to other herbs) in making Kombucha. They point to its benefits as the best medium in which to brew the Kombucha culture because it:

- is rich in minerals and nutrients
- has a high purine content, which the bacteria and yeasts need for metabolism
- produces the highest concentrations of lactic and glucuronic acid.

However, since studying the latest research on the healing properties of green tea, we have begun to use it mainly for our Kombucha tea, thereby producing an even more potent and remarkable health drink. Here is what we have found:-

Despite living in one of the most high-pressured and polluted urban environments on earth, according to a recent study conducted by the National Cancer Institute, Japanese women (who traditionally drink green tea) enjoy the lowest rate of cancer (especially breast cancer), heart disease and have the greatest longevity of all industrialised nations.

According to a 1995 British Medical Journal report: "Japanese green tea has been found to reduce incidence of heart disease". The effect of green tea drinking was analysed in a study of 1371 men in Yoshimi, Japan whose most common beverage was green tea. The results showed that: "The tea reduced the incidence of coronary heart disease, and cardiovascular diseases in general". It was also shown to "improve liver function, therefore providing some protection against liver, colon and lung cancer".

GREEN TEA AS AN ANTI-OXIDANT[1]

One reason why green tea helps prevent cancer and other diseases is because of the polyphenols it contains. These are powerful anti-oxidants, the most potent of which is EGCg. (During fermentation black tea loses certain amounts of beneficial polyphenols including EGCg). The polyphenols fight damage from free radicals responsible for cellular damage caused by toxic chemicals and air pollution implicated in a host of diseases. Victims of the atom bomb were known to have drunk green tea to help remove radiation effects from their bodies.

GREEN TEA AS A CANCER PREVEN-TATIVE[2]

Green tea is believed to help in all three stages of cancer:

- stops tumours forming
- slows their growth
- prevents the growth of cancerous cells in the body

GREEN TEA LOWERS THE RISK OF CARDIOVASCULAR DISEASE[3]

Many heart attacks are caused by an accumulation of plaque on artery walls which block the flow of blood through coronary arteries. Green tea fights heart disease in two very important ways:

- blocks platelet 'clumping'
- significantly lowers cholesterol

EGCg acts similarly to aspirin in helping to prevent blood clotting, but does not irritate the stomach as aspirin can.

Further studies have shown that drinking green tea helps:

- maintain moderate levels of blood sugar
- protect the skin against cancer
- provide a large amount of essential zinc which is required in pregnancy
- prevent tooth decay - (even just rinsing the mouth with green tea after a meal helps)
- combat the causes of high blood pressure by metabolising cholesterol
- prevent premature ageing and strokes

If you have a dilemma on whether to use black or green tea as the preferred medium for Kombucha tea we would recommend that you use *both*. Use black and green tea mixed together in the proportion of say 1:1 - 1:3. Or, try using green or black on their own in alternate brews - interchanging when you feel like it. This way, you will get the best of all worlds, your culture and Kombucha tea brew will be well and happy - and so will you.

Q - Can I use decaffeinated tea?
A - It is best to use unprocessed tea, but some people who are unable to take caffeine have reported success with decaffeinated.

Q - Does any particular type of tea start the fermenting process off quicker than others?
A - Rooibosch Tea (from South Africa), available from health food or delicatessen shops, we have been told cuts a day or so off brewing time and offers a pleasant subtle flavour which is very beneficial mixed in equal parts with green tea.

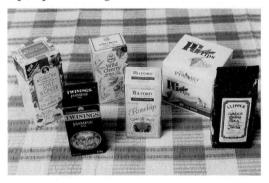

Fig. 23: *A selection of teas: ordinary (fermented), green (unfermented) and herbal*

HERBS

Tea is a herb and research shows that a base of green or black tea is better for the health of the culture and for the quality of Kombucha tea long-term. Other herbs may also be used to impart their medicinal benefits, but it is recommended that you use them *in addition* to tea, either green or black, rather than in place of it.

The main points to bear in mind when using herbs are:

- avoid herbs that contain volatile oils such as; peppermint, fennel, lavender, rosemary, sage and, of course Earl Grey tea, which contains bergamot oil to give it its distinctive flavour. Oils create difficulty in the metabolism and formation of new cultures.

- harvest any herbs you use when their medicinal properties are at their highest, making sure that they are dry and free from rain or dew.

- the herbs must be dried properly in a warm, dry, well-ventilated and shaded place, away from direct sunlight (never use a microwave oven).

- they must be stored well to ensure that they don't develop any mould, risking contamination of the Kombucha brew. Airtight dark containers are good. If clear glass jars are used, they must be kept in a cupboard, as exposure to light causes deterioration of their medicinal properties. Never store in plastic; it encourages condensation.

As a general rule, use twice the amount of herbs to that of tea in the Kombucha recipe. A selection of herbs that can be used are: hawthorn, elderflower, dandelion, nettle, raspberry, strawberry and blackberry leaves.

Harald Tietze, a herbal grower and Kombucha expert, recommends that until you are more experienced with Kombucha brewing that you begin with using herbs that don't grow close to the ground such as elderflower, hawthorn and raspberry leaves, because those that do are more susceptible to bacteria and germs. While many spores are killed at boiling point, some will only be destroyed after prolonged boiling. Tietze goes into the+ use of herbs and their medicinal properties in some detail in his book, *Kombucha - Miracle Fungus: The Essential Handbook.* (*See* "Recommended Reading")

NB: Several coordinators of the Kombucha Tea Network UK recommend that beginners making Kombucha initially stick to using either black or green tea only until they are fully initiated and accustomed to making Kombucha tea well. (This is to reduce the risk of contamination of your Kombucha from poorly dried herbs.) It is then possible to experiment using herbs. Start with commercially sold ones from a reputable source before moving on to home grown and dried ones.

Our favourite Kombucha tea drink using herbs uses equal portions of green tea and dried elderflowers. This makes a beautifully light drink with a lovely bouquet and sparkle. We were told by a wine maker that this would be an excellent choice because elderflower contains an abundance of natural yeasts in its flower heads, which is why it makes a wonderful, sparkling 'Elderflower Champagne'.

Q - What about adding fruits to Kombucha?
A - We have used both dried and fresh fruits in Kombucha and find they make a very pleasant addition to our repertoire. A younger palate will often find Kombucha made with a dried fruit tea or with some fruit cordial added much more acceptable. (For further ideas on using herbs, dried and fresh fruits in Kombucha brewing *see* Chap. 13, "Kombucha Recipes and Other Uses")

WHY WHITE SUGAR, AND CAN HONEY OR OTHER SUGARS BE USED?

Q - I am very health-conscious - do I have to use white sugar?
A - Many health-conscious people are surprised to be told to use refined white sugar in making Kombucha tea and ask whether there is an alternative;

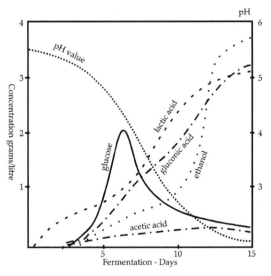

Fig. 24: Conversion of sugar into glucose and then into organic acids. Temperature determines how long this takes. ("Lebensmittelrunschau", 1987)

KOMBUCHA NEEDS SUGAR

Just as we need sugar in order to survive, the Kombucha culture requires sugar and energy, in addition to the minerals and nitrogen it gets from tea, in order for the process of metabolism to take place. The fungus cannot provide its own, therefore you have to provide sugar for it. Sugar is used in assimilation and respiration for most of the fermentation, and during its course is broken down and transformed into acids, vitamins, minerals, enzymes and carbon dioxide. Sugar is also involved in the propagation of the Kombucha culture. At the end of the fermentation period, if done correctly, the sugar will have been virtually all converted and will therefore have been rendered harmless.

Various sugars need to be looked at in order to establish which is better to use for the Kombucha fermentation:

- Household Sugar (granulated) - is refined white sugar and is called sucrose.

- Brown Sugar - most brown sugars, generally considered a more healthy choice than white, are only refined white sugar which has got its colour from a small amount of caramel or molasses added to it.

- Unrefined Brown Sugar - this is raw sugar and has a very strong flavour.

- Raw Cane Sugar - is made mostly into refined white sugar with the remainder steam-heated and sold as pure cane sugar.

- Pure Cane Sugar - is a healthier alternative to granulated white sugar and contains vitamins, minerals and trace elements etc.

In tests using both unrefined brown sugar and raw cane sugar in the Kombucha fermentation the following results were found:

- The solution was dark and cloudy
- The taste was quite unpleasant
- A poorly-formed culture had formed
- There was more yeast sediment
- It contained fewer health-giving organic acids

We decided from this, and from other research and information, that unrefined or raw brown sugar was not suitable for the Kombucha fermentation. Refined white sugar - either granulated or pure cane sugar - is preferable because:

- It is transformed during the fermentation process

- It provides a good nutrient solution for the metabolism of the Kombucha tea

- A healthy culture forms on which to propagate further

- It produces a beverage high in organic acids

- It makes a good and palatable drink

Q - Can honey or malt be used instead of white sugar?
A - Many people choose to use honey in daily use as an alternative sweetener to sugar. Many experts believe that we don't need any added sugars in our diet at all and, if well balanced, will contain all the natural sugars sufficient for our body's needs.

HONEY
Basically honey is composed of around 80% of two simple sugars: glucose and levulose (fructose) and the body is able to assimilate these sugars easily because the bee has already converted them. Since glucose is absorbed directly into the blood it is a quick source of energy.

The requirements of the micro-organism in Kombucha are of prime importance with regards sugar and is not to be regarded as a sweetener. So we need to find out what is best for its main functions and not just for our own preference. While honey is known to have a beneficial bacteriostatic effect on the body, *certain aromatic substances and volatile oils it contains will repress and destroy bacteria and micro-organisms* which are essential in the whole fermentation process of Kombucha.

Some people who are determined to prove that honey can be used, have managed to produce a Kombucha tea that looks good and tastes pleasant. Unfortunately they have not had the properties of their brew or the fungus analysed long-term. It has been found in research that modifications and mutations can suddenly appear and alter the organism after a period of time using honey. Our advice, therefore, is to heed the researchers and doctors, many of whom have tried and would have preferred to use honey if they could, but who have concluded that Kombucha *prefers refined* white sugar - cane or granulated - in the fermentation process.

As Alick is a beekeeper and we have a plentiful supply, we enjoy the full unadulterated health benefits of honey in our diet, but would suggest that you too use refined sugar when making your Kombucha tea.

MALT

Research found that malt could produce reasonably good cultures but the Kombucha beverage lacked strength in organic acids.

WATER - WHY CHEMICAL FREE?

Q - Why is there so much emphasis placed on using filtered water in making Kombucha tea?

A - Water is fundamental to life itself; after all the human body is composed of as much as 70% water and cannot sustain life long without it. Our veins and arteries are like natural rivers coursing through our bodies taking nutrients wherever they are needed. It is obvious then, that pure, sparkling, 'live' highland spring water will do you much more good than the adulterated, chemically treated water that comes out of most of our taps.

You have to ask yourself - why are more and more people getting ill with cancer, Alzheimer's disease, immune deficiency diseases such as Chronic Fatigue Syndrome, allergies, eczema and asthma? And why are some of these affecting our children at a younger age than ever before? Our whole body's system is becoming weakened and more toxic due to the pollutants and chemicals that we absorb over a long period of time, some of which comes from the chemically treated water that we drink.

THE CHEMICAL COCKTAILS ADDED TO OUR WATER SUPPLY

Water that comes out of our taps is often cloudy, and can have the familiar smell of the chlorine which is added to kill bacteria, in addition to other chemicals. Some authorities also add aluminium sulphate and fluorides, the long term effects of which are causing controversy which has not yet been resolved. Chemicals such as nitrates, pesticides and herbicides which are poured onto our farmland in huge amounts, leach into the underground water table, as do the chemical effluent toxic substances and industrial wastes which also pollute rivers. These, in combination with chemicals used in filtration plants to recycle water, the heavy metals in old lead pipes and the toxic substances released from new plastic replacement ones make an unpleasant cocktail for our precious bodies to cope with. It must be said that some water authorities are trying harder than others to reduce some of these problems. Veins and arteries, which carry nutrients, will also carry the chemicals that we absorb into our bloodstream affecting **all** areas of the body. Our immune systems become weakened, we may develop allergies, function less well and can become ill. You have a right to know what is in your water, so some judicious enquiries would be a good idea!

BOTTLED WATER - IS IT AN ALTERNATIVE?

Bottled water is often recommended for Kombucha tea making. However, recent research has shown that most bottled waters *are not safe*.[4] Bottled water companies do not have to meet the same safety standards as the major water authorities. No information is usually required on the presence of pesticides and herbicides, and they need to test fewer than 25% of the substances that are required of the water authorities. For example, excessive mineral contamination is usually not monitored.

The other factor is that bottled water, which is usually sold in plastic bottles, sits in warehouses and on supermarket shelves, developing bacteria. This, and the toxicity of the plastic, do not make it a good alternative source for Kombucha tea. (*See Footnote 6*)

THE NEED TO FILTER OUR WATER

Chlorine which is added to water supplies to kill harmful bacteria will, unfortunately, also affect the millions of friendly bacteria in Kombucha.[5] That is why the water you use for brewing your Kombucha tea should be filtered. This can be done by using a cartridge and jug, or a system plumbed in under the sink. Jug filters will remove chlorine from water and make it taste better. However, only the best quality water filters will remove aluminium, bacteria and heavy metals, like lead, along with organic pollutants such as herbicides and pesticides. Water filtering systems do vary, so we would advise you to do your own research and always to buy the best you can afford. (*See* "Resource Section and Suppliers")

BOILING WATER

If you don't have a water filter, make sure that you boil your water for at least five minutes to dispel chlorine and to destroy bacteria if it is well, spring or 'untreated' water.

MAKING WATER COME ALIVE AGAIN!

We believe that the water we drink is rendered lifeless and without 'life-force' due to the various chemical treatments and recycling processes applied to it. When natural spring water (not from a bottle) is tested with a dowsing pendulum, it spins to the right (clockwise), showing that the water has a positive life-force. When normal tap or bottled water is tested, the pendulum spins to the left (anti-clockwise) indicating that it has no life-force. In other words, it is biologically dead! We believe in re-activating our water by turning it into a clockwise spin, and do this by putting it through a 'Spiraliser'. This is a very simple and cheap method which uses a tin-plated copper spiral inside a funnel, creating a vortex motion. *All* our water is put through this process which we believe transforms its energy state and changes the taste. Kombucha (and cheap wine) that tastes a little sharp can even have its flavour improved by 'spiralising' it. Putting all your liquids through the vortex could help you re-energise, your animals and plants too. (*See* "Resource Section and Suppliers")

THE USE OF VINEGAR AS THE FIRST 'STARTER'

Q- What is the purpose of using vinegar in the beginning with my first batch of Kombucha?
A- The addition of an acid 'starter' at the beginning of the fermentation process is to increase acidity and activate bacteria in the medium and also to act as protection against unfavourable micro-organisms.

Q - Does vinegar have to be used with every batch?
A - No, cider or wine vinegar is only used in the first batch you make if no 'mother' starter brew (the actual Kombucha tea) is available. After this the 'mother' Kombucha tea only is used as a starter. If vinegar was used on its own every time or in addition to the 'mother' starter, it would make the Kombucha tea too acidic and vinegary.

You can however use some cider or wine vinegar as a 'kick-start' (as we call it) if the ferment seems to need a boost and the beverage has become, or is still, a bit flat with resulting thin cultures. Other causes should be looked at also e.g. insufficient heat etc.

Q - Can malt or distilled vinegar be used as a starter, or do I have to use Cider or wine vinegar and why?
A - Always use organic cider or wine vinegar. In the USA (though not in Europe) the FDA permits distilled vinegar to be made from petroleum rather than food-grade products! So keep those vinegars for washing windows only.

Q - Can alcohol be used instead of vinegar or Kombucha tea as a 'starter'?
A - The addition of alcohol at the beginning of Kombucha fermentation has been experimented with over previous decades, but has been deemed unnecessary. The addition of alcohol activates bacteria (as vinegar and the Kombucha tea 'mother' starter also does) and a shot of rum, sherry, port or cognac added was according to Lindner (1917) - to make it possible for the bacteria to begin making acetic acid right away, in case the yeasts had not yet developed.

With the addition of alcohol, the layer of mucilage is more transparent. This explains why, in the acidic environment, the forming culture is more clear and gelatinous at first as the bacteria have a head start on the yeasts, which come in later to form the denser culture and bring it together.

Q - What happens if I have used vinegar that is very old and may have gone off?
A - Always play safe with Kombucha and get a new fungus plus a new bottle of organic, cider or wine vinegar.

HEATING METHODS FOR KOMBUCHA TEA BREWING

Q - Which is the best heat source for making Kombucha tea?
A - There are many different heat methods for brewing Kombucha. Here is a selection for you to explore:

THE AIRING CUPBOARD OR HOT LINEN CLOSET

Most people find that brewing Kombucha in the airing cupboard works very well for them though there are certain important considerations to take into account:

- Is the hot water tank well insulated, which will mean that more heat is retained in the water, leaving less to warm the cupboard?

- Is the hot water system on a time-control which turns the heat on and off periodically, leading to large temperature fluctuations during fermentation? Temperature drops can be reduced by lagging or insulating your vessel with a large folded towel that will help retain some warmth

- How far do you have to travel within the home to get from the kitchen to the airing cupboard? Some people find this journey difficult if it involves negotiating stairs while carrying a container of liquid.

If the temperature is right (fluctuations are not extreme) and the journey poses no problem then this method is certainly the best and the cheapest. Remember to leave the door slightly ajar to allow some air to circulate (and don't forget to wedge it, if you have a cat, to stop it getting in, causing it and your Kombucha problems!)

THE BOILER ROOM

This can be another ideal place for Kombucha fermentation - though boiler rooms vary in their suitability. As long as yours is clean, warm and dry, it will be fine. If it is a glory hole full of junk, then forget it!

ELECTRIC HEATING TRAYS

These are ideal, being specially made for brewing. They are sold in four different sizes, depending on how much Kombucha tea you want to make, and include one for the Continuous Fermentation Method. (*See* "Resource Section and Suppliers")
The advantages of using a heating tray are:

- It has a low wattage and is thermostatically controlled to maintain the correct constant temperature for fermentation.

- It cuts down considerably on brewing time because it provides 24-hour continuous heat. As a consequence you can make more Kombucha Tea.

- The cultures produced are of a good quality.

- It is very convenient because you can site your tray and container on a kitchen work top, near to water, kettle and other ingredients.

NB: Because of its extra efficiency in providing 24-hour heat, it may be necessary, when using a heating tray, to add some extra water to make up for some evaporation. For the 2-litre/4-pint batch brewing method we add $1/2$-pint of extra water. For large quantities it isn't so necessary.

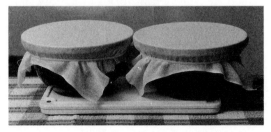

Fig. 25: Two 2-litre bowls on an electric heating tray

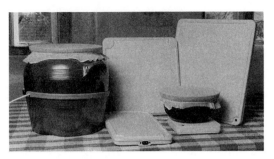

Fig.26: An electric heating belt and four sizes of electric heating trays

ELECTRIC HEATING BELT

This is a circular, soft, rubber adjustable belt designed to wrap around a large home-brewing beer barrel and is only suitable for large fermentation containers.

SUBMERSIBLE HEATER

This is normally sold for heating fish tanks, but some people have written in to say that it can work well for large containers of fermenting Kombucha.

A GREENHOUSE HEATER

When we first started to make lots of Kombucha tea and cultures to send out to people through the Kombucha Network, we fitted a cupboard with slatted shelves and used a simple 60 watt cylindrical greenhouse heater in the bottom connected to an electric adapter with thermostatic controls to regulate the temperature.

With the addition of a simple thermometer to monitor the environment, this works very well. You can purchase these greenhouse heaters sold in several different sizes and wattages, depending on the space you want to heat, from plumbing wholesalers, so they are worth investigating locally.

THE COOKIE TIN AND LIGHT BULB SOLUTION

We have a friend whose handyman thought of this (and full marks for inventiveness and cheapness). She had a small empty cupboard in her living room that she wanted to use for her Kombucha tea brewing. The handyman secured a light bulb in the centre of an upturned large cookie tin (in which he'd made a hole) to the roof of the cup-

board. The reflection of the light on the metal created sufficient heat for the fermentation, and she became a proud and successful Kombucha brewer. The only drawback was the fruity aroma from the fermenting Kombucha tea in her living room. She didn't find it unpleasant, but it was certainly a talking point with visitors.

NB: It is obviously important to practise safety when dealing with electricity and liquids, so, please, no flimsy constructions. Be sure you know what you are doing - or get an expert.

Whichever heating system you use, we recommend that you use a thermometer to check the temperature. This will ensure that you make a success of your Kombucha tea brewing. Simple thermometers are quite cheap and well worth investing in (available from most hardware stores or *see* "Resource Section and Suppliers")

BREWING CONTAINERS - WHAT IS THE RIGHT TYPE?

Q - I have a big glass jar, will this be OK to use for Kombucha brewing?
A - The container needs to have a wide opening at the top as the fermenting Kombucha brew needs a good supply of oxygen to work effectively. A bowl is much better than a long tall jar with a small opening.

Q - What type of container is best for my Kombucha brewing, and can I use plastic?
A - Your container needs to be made of a material that is non-toxic and will not have chemicals released into the acidic medium. The recommended ones are made of:- glass, china, high-glaze porcelain or enamel (unchipped). 'Pyrex' glass bowls are good and easily obtained in most hardware stores across the world. Use the 3-litre/6-pint size for the batch brewing method recipe in this book.

Materials which are *not advised* include: aluminium, plastics (even food-grade), ceramic, some coloured glass and lead crystal glass. The reason is that acids in Kombucha, notably acetic acid, will leach toxins from these types of containers into the beverage.

Aluminium - is widely advised against. It is common knowledge that once a can of tomatoes is opened, the contents must be poured out immediately, because the action of air with the acids in the tomatoes will leach aluminium from the tin into the produce. As a general rule, all aluminium cooking utensils should be banished from the kitchen as this metal is detrimental to health. Research has also linked aluminium with Alzheimer's disease.

Plastics - There is much to be aware of in our modern over-use of plastics. A number of companies have developed a wide range of synthetic oil-based products under umbrella patents for commercial use. One of these products, PVC. (polyvinyl chloride), is now used in an enormous range of applications including kitchen and household products. No long-term research has ever been carried out on the possible systemic effects. There is evidence however that PVC. and chemical compounds used to make plastic more stable and impact - resistant are potential carcinogens and may disrupt normal hormonal function. Other dysfunctions that may result are impotence, birth defects, menstrual disorders and disruption of the endocrine system.[6]

We want you to make a health drink, not a cocktail of toxins, so it is important that Kombucha is made in a container that is suitable for the purpose, so definitely *no plastics*. We would also seriously suggest that we all look at our present uses of plastics in food preparation and storage and in the home as well. We have banished all plastic containers from our kitchen.

Ceramic and Lead Glass Crystal - both these products use metals either in the glaze or in the contents of the glass, which will leach into the Kombucha beverage and are not recommended. Also beware of coloured glass and cheap glazed earthenware.

QUESTIONS ABOUT FERMENTATION

Q - How long will it take me to make Kombucha tea?
A - It only takes about 10-15 minutes for one or more batch brewing bowls per week and it takes even less time using the Continuous Fermentation Method (*See* Chapter 5, "How to Brew Kombucha Successfully")

Q - If I have put the Kombucha fungus into hot liquid will it kill it?
A - Yes, definitely!

Q - Is it OK if I have left my tea to brew for more than fifteen minutes before adding it to the Kombucha starter?
A - Yes, but as in making tea, the flavour strengthens and becomes slightly more bitter which will affect your Kombucha brew. Everything you do in the whole process will in some way affect the overall taste of your Kombucha tea.

Q - Can anything be done to hasten the start of the brewing process?
A - Don't let the sweet tea brew you have made get cold. As soon as the temperature of the liquid has cooled to about blood or room temperature add the 'starter' liquid and the fungus.

Q - Why does the fermenting beverage require oxygen?
A - The Kombucha culture requires oxygen for metabolic processes to take place and would starve without it.

Q - Can I brew more or less than the recipe says?
A - More - yes; just measure all the ingredients proportionally as in the batch brewing recipe. Less - no; the recipe doesn't work well scaled down, and the resulting beverage becomes too strong and acidic.

Q - I don't have an airing cupboard; does this matter?
A - No, but you will have to find some other warm situation for the fermentation to be successful. If you have nothing available in the home then we suggest you obtain an electric heating tray. Most people who re-

port failure in brewing Kombucha have insufficient heat.

Q - If I have forgotten to add the 'starter' can it be added a few days later?
A - Yes, it is not ideal, but add this onto the brewing time.

Q - Does it matter that I haven't left it to ferment long enough, as it still tastes sweet?
A - It doesn't matter as long as sugar doesn't adversely affect you, though the beverage won't have as many health-giving properties as when all the sugar has been allowed to convert fully into organic acids, vitamins and minerals. It will also not be an effective 'starter' for your next batch of Kombucha so you will need to add 1-2 tablespoons of cider or wine vinegar to compensate as well as the 'starter'.

Q - All the sweetness has gone but it still tastes flat. Why?
A - Check that your brewing temperature is warm enough and that the Kombucha 'starter' has been added. Try adding 1-2 tablespoons of cider or wine vinegar as a 'kick-start' with your next batch. If the Kombucha tea still doesn't improve, then get another new healthy culture and start again.

Q - What is the sediment left on the bottom of my brewqing bowl?
A - These are old yeast cells and can be left in the bottom of the container if you are making a new batch immediately. Rinse the container after every few fermentations or each time you brew if you prefer.

Q - Nothing seems to be happening, what's gone wrong?
A - By about the third day of fermentation, you should see signs of a thin film beginning to cover the surface of the liquid. If you don't see this, check that your temperature is high enough. Most slow or under-performing cultures do not have enough warmth. Also, did you add the starter liquid? If you think that you have done everything correctly, sit tight and leave well alone. If by the seventh day nothing is happening, try a new culture.

Q - The pH is not reaching at least 3 on the pH strip.
A - Leave the brew to ferment longer. Also check that your brewing temperature is high enough and your ingredients are correct. It can take 2-3 fermentations at the beginning to obtain a vibrant Kombucha tea strong enough to reach the ideal pH of 2·6-3, after which you will probably be successful.

Q - The electric heating tray seems too hot.
A - The temperature of the tray is designed to give 9°C (16°F) above room temperature, the average room being 15°C (58°F), therefore giving an ideal liquid temperature of 24°C (74°F) for Kombucha brewing. Remember, the liquid in your bowl will not be the same as the temperature of the actual heating tray!

Q - The tray seems warm, but fermentation doesn't seem to be working very well.
A - It may have to do with the base of your bowl. If it has a very thick rim, air may be trapped between the bowl and the tray, creating a 'double-glazing' effect. It is better to use a container with a shallow base rim.

Q - Our Kombucha tea evaporates quite a lot during fermentation, what can be done about this?
A - With higher temperatures, especially on electric heating trays and with heating systems in a cupboard turned up high there may be a certain amount of evaporation. If you find that this is happening with your batch brewing bowl then add ¼-½ -pint of extra water at the beginning to compensate, (there is no need to add any extra tea or sugar though).

Q - What is the fruity smell given off during fermentation?
A - This is a familiar smell of Kombucha brewing and develops after a few days into fermentation. It then eases off again when the beverage is almost ready.

Q - What happens if my Kombucha slows down and doesn't seem to be working so well?
A - How long have you been using your 'mother' culture? For it to perform at full strength, you should use a culture 6-8 times

and then replace it with a new one. Poor performance can also be due to a change in the weather or sudden drop in temperature. This can be especially noticeable in autumn/fall before your heating goes on.

Q - If I stop the fermentation too soon, can I restart it and continue?
A - Yes, Kombucha can take it, though it's not ideal as it prefers continuity and little disruption.

Q - There is a film like scum forming over the liquid in my brew, is this normal?
A - It is almost certainly the new culture forming on the surface, so leave well alone. However, if it still looks like scum after 7-10 days, then it is not working properly - usually because of a lack of warmth during fermentation or incorrect ingredients.

Q - A thick jelly-like thing has formed on top of the liquid. What is it?
A - Congratulations, a new healthy culture has been produced and all is well.

Q - Does the new offspring form on top of the original culture or underneath it?
A - Always on top, it grows over the whole surface of the liquid and on top of the mother culture (if it is floating).

Q - What are the whitish-looking blobs on the surface of the liquid?
A - This is the second stage of the new culture forming. The process can vary, sometimes forming smaller or bigger blobs that gradually join together to form a whole mass, at other times it can grow more uniformly and evenly.

Q - If Russian peasants brewed Kombucha tea in their kitchens, why all the fuss about hygiene?
A - Kitchens don't have to be clinically clean, but a certain level of sensible hygiene is important when handling any fresh food and it is certainly very important for successful Kombucha fermentation too.

Q - Can I put my fermentation bowl in a spare room or cupboard?
A - Only if you provide some form of heat and the cupboard is clean with sufficient air circulation.

Q - Does smoke affect Kombucha?
A - There are reports that tobacco smoke in the same room has killed a culture or made it go mouldy. A small amount of wood smoke can be tolerated, though it would probably affect the taste - and we aren't sure about joss sticks - though they too would certainly flavour the Kombucha tea if regularly used in the same room as fermentation!

Q - Can plants be kept anywhere in the same room?
A - It is not advisable to have plants near the fungus, as their spores can transfer and cause mould to develop on the culture.

Q - Our house is damp; will I still be able to brew?
A - It may be difficult. Unfortunately spores are invisible to the naked eye and can travel very easily. Find the driest part of the house and have a go. Your best bet is to use an electric heating tray. If that fails, maybe you should take steps to solve your damp problems - or move house so that you can make your Kombucha tea successfully!

QUESTIONS ABOUT KOMBUCHA TEA

Q - Can I drink the beverage as soon as it is ready?
A - It is better to leave it for at least 3-5 days before drinking to give the Kombucha tea a fuller, rounder flavour, but this is not essential. Some people believe that the beverage tastes even better after a few weeks of storage.

Q - If I put the live beverage in the refrigerator, will this make it less active?
A - No, the fermentation process slows down almost to a halt but the 'live' qualities of the beverage are still very much present.

Q - If the drink is too sour for me, can I add more sugar to the recipe?
A - This is not the answer. Stop the fermentation process earlier, just at the point where the sweet taste has gone and before it has begun to turn sour/vinegary. The recipe has been worked out exactly to enable the right amount of sugar in the given volume of liq-

uid to be converted, resulting in a beverage which contains the highest possible proportion of all its health-giving properties.

You can always add some fruit juice to the Kombucha tea if it is a bit sour to make it more palatable. If it has turned completely to Kombucha vinegar, do not drink the full recommended amount. You could safely drink only 1-2 tablespoons, though, in some water or fruit juice.

Q - Why does my Kombucha tea foam when I pour it into a bottle?
A - The foam is caused by carbonation - that is, carbon dioxide released through exposure to air - and is quite normal. It is a sign of a healthy beverage. Sometimes it is quite fizzy and frothy when poured, at other times less so.

Q - Why is it sometimes cloudy?
A - This is caused by the development of yeasts during the fermentation process, which can be greater in some brewing batches than in others. It will also show when a continuous fermentation container needs to be cleaned out.

Q - Can I buy Kombucha tea commercially?
A - Yes, it is becoming more widely available and we expect it will soon be in most wholefood stores. Bottled Kombucha needs to be cold-stored to prevent it from fermenting further at room temperature and turning sour.

Q - Can I sell my Kombucha beverage?
A - It is illegal to sell any food or drink commercially without inspections by the relevant health departments who ensure that all standards of hygiene are being met. This is necessary for your own protection.

Q - Kombucha reminds me of cider vinegar; does it have the same properties?
A - Vinegar has a long history of being used in a healing capacity and apple cider has been much praised in modern times. Many of the organisms and biochemical reactions in Kombucha are similar to those in cider vinegar, and have some comparable healing and cleansing properties. Kombucha is even more potent and beneficial than apple cider vinegar because of the unique and wide range of organic acids it contains. If your

Kombucha tea tastes like vinegar then it has been left too long to ferment, so stop it earlier. You can however use this mature Kombucha in many ways. (*See* Chapter 13, "Kombucha Recipes and Other Uses")

ALL ABOUT
THE KOMBUCHA FUNGUS

You must remember that the Kombucha fungus is a living organism and should be treated with due respect by ensuring that it always has an adequate nutrient solution and supply of oxygen to keep it well and happy.

Q - What exactly is it and how does it work?
A - Kombucha is a living organism, a symbiosis of yeasts and bacteria, and when added to a nutrient solution of tea and sugar and placed in a warm environment, the fermentation and oxidation processes commence like a little chemical factory at work. It feeds on the sugars and converts them into a nutritious 'food' drink, Kombucha tea, which contains a wide range of organic acids, vitamins, enzymes and minerals which are essential for good health.

Q - Why is my new culture a different colour from the one I was given?
A - All cultures vary slightly in colour. If your newly formed culture is a different colour from the one that you were given, it is just that a different tea has been used. The fungus is like a sponge and picks up its colour from the liquid. If black tea is used it will be a beige/brown, if green tea it will be aler, more whitish in colour.

Q - The culture I was sent is smaller than my brewing bowl, is this OK and will this piece grow at all?
A - It doesn't matter what size or shape your starter 'mother' culture is. A piece easuring 3-4 inches is usual and sufficient to start a batch brewing bowl of 2-litres/ 4-pints in volume. This 'mother' culture *will always remain the same size*. However, the new culture forms *on the surface of the liquid* during fermentation and will always grow to the size and shape of your container.

Q - Should I start my second batch of Kombucha with the original fungus or use my new 'offspring'?
A - You can use either. The original or any 'mother' culture can be used up to 6-8 times. If your new 'offspring' has not grown as thick as the 'mother', use the original piece until you start producing healthier, thicker ones.

Q - Can I give my original piece of starter culture away to a new Kombucha brewer if I have only used it once?
A - Yes, if you are satisfied that you are producing substantial new cultures - but always keep at least one good back-up culture for yourself in case anything ever goes wrong.

Q - Do I have to use a bigger starter culture if I am brewing a large quantity?
A - Yes, it is wise to increase the starter culture size if you can. Many books say that it doesn't matter, but we have found that it does make some difference; by saving fermentation time plus it makes a better quality drink if you scale the size up accordingly.

Q - Can I use the whole culture that has formed from my first batch as a starter, or do I only have to use a smaller piece?
A - You can use the whole or smaller piece, it doesn't matter as either will work well.

Q - Does it matter if the fungus has got holes or a tear in it?
A - No, not at all. It may only affect the look of the new one forming; i.e. it may be a bit patchy in thickness (but not always - it could form perfectly). It doesn't really matter what shape it is, as long as it is a healthy piece of culture. To be sure of obtaining a completely smooth culture, if this is your goal, let it fall to the bottom of the bowl and weight it down with a clean object, so that a new unconnected culture forms on the top of the liquid.

Q - What are the brown stringy bits, like tendrils, on the underside of the fungus is this mould?
A - No, they are dead yeast cells and are absolutely harmless.

Q - Should I wash the fungus before use?
A - There is no reason to do so, but, if you do, please don't use tap water. We usually give out clean funguses with no brown, stringy tendrils on them, to put off new brewers!

With clean hands as you are removing the culture from the ferment, simply rinse the brown bits off into the liquid - (this gets strained off pouring into bottles anyway) or rinse separately using some spare Kombucha tea.

Q - Can I eat the fungus and can I give pieces to animals?
A - The Kombucha fungus is very concentrated, tough and rubbery in texture and not particularly palatable on its own. However, it can be chopped up into salads. Some animals, especially dogs, will take small pieces on their own, or the fungus can be cut up and mixed into its food.

Q - Can I use a thin fungus to start a new batch of Kombucha?
A - A thin culture from a weak brew is not a good idea to use. If this is all that your first ferment(s) has produced then use the original piece of 'starter' fungus as well as the thin fungus to start off the next batch. Do this several times if necessary until your Kombucha brew, and resulting funguses, grow thicker, healthy and strong.

Q - The piece of culture I was given is over half an inch thick. Is this OK to use and should I expect my new offspring to be just as thick?
A - It will probably have come from someone who has been brewing in larger quantities where the cultures grows thicker or has been left longer than usual in fermentation. It is perfectly all right to use, but don't expect your new 'offspring' to be as thick if you are using the quantity contained in the batch brewing method. Alternatively it may have come from a very healthy beverage - in which case be prepared for surprises. It could also have come from someone who has been using a container with a smaller liquid surface area which would produce smaller, thicker cultures.

Q - I can't separate the new culture from the 'mother'?

A - The new culture that forms usually separates very easily from the 'mother', but sometimes they fuse together. Simply snip them apart with scissors that have been sterilised in boiling water for a few minutes and allowed to cool. Older cultures do fuse together however if they are not separated with each ferment, and are allowed to pile up one on top of another.

Q - How do I know if my fungus is healthy?

A - By obtaining it from a responsible organisation or from someone whom you would consider to be an intelligent, clean and caring person, capable of brewing Kombucha correctly and responsibly. Ask the donor questions from the information on page 30.

Q - The culture pulls apart into pieces very easily in my hands; is this normal?

A - If the fungus is actually falling apart, then, no, it is not healthy and we would suggest that you get a new healthy culture from a different source.

Q - What can I do with my old funguses that need retiring?

A - Put them spread out on the compost heap for preference if you have one. They have given good service, thank them and let them go. You can also dig them into the garden chopped up around acid loving plants, but not if your soil is already on the acid side. If you don't have a proper compost heap or garden, then they have to be garbaged.

Q - What can I do with my good spare funguses?

A - If you are convinced that they are healthy and worthy of passing on, you could advertise them in a local wholefood shop or health centre. Be prepared to give advice though, and have some of your time taken up nursing new brewers along. Most Kombucha networks will only use cultures from experienced brewers who are known to them, which keeps the standards high.

Q - The new culture has brown patches on the surface; is this OK?

A - It probably means that it has dried out a little and hasn't been in total contact with the liquid. If you see this happening, with clean hands push it under the liquid and check that the fermentation temperature isn't too high.

Q - How do I know if my culture has got mould on it?

A - It will be very visible as a soft or hairy growth on the surface of the culture as can be seen on mouldy food, in colours ranging from green, black, white, grey or orange. If you discover mould, you should discard the fungus and the brew. Start with all sterilised equipment, a fresh culture and find the cause.

Q - Can I use the culture again if it has got mould on it?

A - No, definitely not. You will need to sterilise all your equipment and the environment thoroughly and obtain a new culture. If it happens again you will have to think of looking carefully at all your ingredients, e.g. tea and herbs to see if there is any possibility of contamination or brewing in another situation.

Q - I have read that you can wash a culture with mould on with vinegar or lemon juice to clean it, does this work?

A - No. Some publications suggest this, but we disagree entirely with this practice. Washing puts the spores in a solution where they are then able to spread even further over the culture and beyond. We don't know anyone who has found success with this method and mould has always returned in the next fermentation.

Q - Can I drink the liquid from a batch that has a mouldy culture on top?

A - No, definitely not. It is dangerous to drink Kombucha tea contaminated with mould (*aspergillus*) which produces water-soluble toxins, and can result in illness. We wouldn't dream of eating or drinking any other mouldy food or drink and there is no difference with Kombucha tea.

Q - Is it OK to cut the fungus with scissors? I have heard that you mustn't let metal come into contact with it?
A - It is OK to use scissors, especially if they are made of stainless steel, as contact with the fungus is too brief to do it any harm. Sterilise the scissors first though. Being told to take off your rings while handling the culture is also inappropriate advice.

Q - Why do my baby funguses grow thinner in the winter?
A - The fungus is affected by changing weather when the heating may be off and the temperature drops at night, and especially between the late summer seasons, autumn and winter. Funguses seem to grow better in spring and summer, especially during the hottest months when they work at a greater metabolic rate.

Q - My funguses sometimes develop bubbles or have a warty appearance. Is this normal?
A - It happens usually because the heat is high or more carbon dioxide is being produced in this fermentation. The culture will still be perfectly all right to use though.

Q - Can I let my funguses pile up and not separate them?
A - The ones underneath will gradually die off. The funguses may also become invasive, taking up too much volume or space, especially in the Batch Brewing Method. It is better to separate them after 1-2 fermentations - unless they are on the thin side and need to be used together. If you use a large container, you can probably let your funguses pile up a little longer, cutting a piece off when you need to restart.

Q - How many times can I use the original 'mother' culture?
A - The recommended lifespan of a culture is 6-8 times. The characteristic metabolism of the various micro-organisms on which the therapeutic effect of Kombucha tea is based, can only be carried out by good fresh cultures. If a culture is used too long, the tea will not ferment so well and the resulting drink will be more acidic.

Q - Can the cultures be sent by mail, if so how?
A - Yes. We mail them in thick-gauge plastic bags and use a heat-sealing unit to prevent any liquid escaping or use several zip-lock bags. The culture is like a sponge, so you need to take special care not to send leaky packages in the post. What gets out can also get in, and the liquid can become a channel for contamination.

STORING AND PRESERVING KOMBUCHA

KOMBUCHA TEA

Q - Can Kombucha tea be stored, and if so how long for?
A - When your Kombucha tea is ready it is important to bottle and store it immediately in a cold place to slow the fermentation right down. The refrigerator is ideal, because its temperature virtually stops the fermentation process, thereby preventing the tea from going sour. If you only have enough room for one bottle of Kombucha at a time in the refrigerator, then store the rest in as cool a place as possible, such as a garage or outbuilding. In a warm room, fermentation will continue slowly and gradually turn the Kombucha sour and vinegary. Beware of commercial Kombucha beverage that is displayed out of a refrigerator, as it will probably be sour if it has been there for a week or two.

Q - How long will Kombucha tea keep?
A - Up to 3 months if stored in a cold place. It can even improve with age. After 4 months however we have experienced it going off.

Q - Is there anything I can do to preserve it naturally?
A - We don't think that it is necessary to add any preservative as Kombucha tea stores for 2-3 months very well anyway on its own without anything being added to it. If you do want to try it though we have been advised that adding 1-gram (the tip of a teaspoon) of ascorbic acid when you are bottling, will help to preserve Kombucha tea

longer . Ascorbic acid can be obtained from chemists and drug stores.

Q - How should I store Kombucha; do I only use glass bottles to put my Kombucha tea in or can I use plastic?
A - Always store Kombucha in glass bottles, and never plastic, as again they can easily leach toxins. You can use screw-top caps, filling the bottle right up to the top without an air space to keep in the effervescence, as there is not usually enough carbon dioxide or fizz in the beverage to cause a problem. If you do have a very effervescent Kombucha brew at any time then corking would be a safer method. Once the bottle has been opened it will go flat, but will still taste good.

Q - My stored Kombucha Tea grows a mini culture on top of the liquid, is this normal?
A - Yes, this can occur even with Kombucha that has been stored at a coolish room temperature after 2-3 weeks. It shows that it is a healthy living beverage and simply needs straining off. We made a very successful new batch of Kombucha using one of these healthy little cultures from a stored bottle of Kombucha tea.

Q - What are the small jelly-like things growing in the Kombucha tea stored in the refrigerator?
A - Even with efficient filtering of the fermented liquid, you will not be able to eliminate all yeast and bacteria cells. These stimulate new culture growth, but the process is reduced enormously in the cold environment of the refrigerator. It is a simple process to strain every glass you pour through a small sieve. The jelly bits won't harm you and some people don't even bother to do this. It shows the remarkable nature of the 'live' Kombucha tea health drink.

THE FUNGUS/CULTURE

Q - How can I store my spare funguses and how long will they keep?
A - They will keep for several months stored in a refrigerator covered in a mixture of equal quantities of Kombucha tea and cold sweet tea. Once restarted, the fungus may take 2-3 fermentations to come out of its semi-hibernation state to a stage where it performs fully.

Sometimes, for no apparent reason, your culture may decide not to work so well, so it is always advisable to have a spare one in hand. If you are stockpiling several for a long period of time, strain off this liquid periodically and top up with a fresh mixture. Remember to rotate them, always giving away the oldest one first.

DRYING THE CULTURE

Q - Can I dry the culture and if so how?
A - Cultures can be successfully dried at home but care needs to be taken to make sure that the environmental conditions are good so that unfavourable bacteria do not settle on the cultures during this time. It is a good way of preserving them for very long spells away or for posting a culture to far-off lands. To make a success of it you will need to have the right temperature of 32°C (90°F). At higher temperatures the culture will be damaged and not ferment properly when reconstituted. Never use a microwave oven or direct sunlight.

When dried, the Kombucha culture will look like dried brown leather, but once placed into a nutrient solution it will swell up and the micro-organisms will become active again. In Germany, back in the 1920s, dried Kombucha was reportedly used in the production of imitation leather and was tanned and fashioned into kid gloves. We have also heard that in poor countries dried Kombucha was used to sole shoes, but goodness knows what happened if it rained!

FREEZING THE CULTURE

Q - Can the cultures be frozen or will it harm them?
A - Freeze-drying is a successful method for preserving Kombucha but needs special equipment. If you use your domestic freezer it is very important to do it properly. Your culture must be frozen as fast as possible. If freezing takes place too slowly crystals will form which will damage the Kombucha culture's cells.

Here is how to proceed:

- Switch on the fast-freeze setting of your freezer well in advance so that the culture can be frozen as quickly as possible.
- Place the culture and some fermented Kombucha tea in a suitable container or plastic bag secured at the top.
- Label and freeze.
- When thawing out, place the block of ice containing the culture into some fresh Kombucha beverage and allow to defrost slowly at room temperature.

Please note that your defrosted culture will take longer than usual to fully ferment in the Kombucha tea, as it has been in hibernation. But be patient, because just when you are tempted to give up, thinking that it has probably died in suspended animation, you will begin to see some activity, confirming that your culture is alive and well. It may take several ferments for it to come back into full active service again, but you will be rewarded well for your perseverance.

GOING ON HOLIDAY OR VACATION

Q - What is the best way to keep my Kombucha fungus while I am away on holiday?
A - If you are going away for any length of time, the following method will help your culture survive well:

- Place the fungus in the brewing container and add the usual amount of sweet tea and Kombucha 'starter' beverage.
- Cover with muslin or a fine cotton fabric and secure with elastic.
- Stand the container in a *cool*, clean place where the activity will be slowed down considerably. You can leave it there for several weeks or even months. When you return home simply pour off the liquid and your culture will be ready for use again. It will probably have even produced a fine healthy 'offspring' as a surprise too. The resulting sour beverage won't be drinkable but can be used in the kitchen or bathroom. If it hasn't quite reached becoming vinegar, you could

put it in a warm place to ferment further and turn it into Kombucha vinegar.

Q - I am going on holiday and don't want to stop taking my Kombucha.
A - You can now buy concentrated Kombucha in capsule form, which makes it ideal for travelling. Home-made live Kombucha tea is always best though for the rest of the time, and is also a fraction of the price. (*See* "Resource Section and Suppliers")

Q - Can I take the brew when I travel?
A - Yes, but don't forget it is a living beverage and will continue to ferment, even in a capped bottle at normal temperatures. You could stop the fermentation early, before it is ready and then continue the fermentation when you get to your destination.

Another way is to put your Kombucha tea into cool bags with ice packs, and refrigerate it as soon as you reach your destination. In medieval times.

Japanese warriors used to take a flaskful of Kombucha tea with a culture in it, and then top up with sweet tea as they drank it - an ancient form of the Continuous Fermentation method; you could try that!

REFERENCES

1   *Future Med Catalog,* "Self-Healing Resources"

2   Epidemiological and Experiential Studies on the Antitumor Activity by Green Tea Extracts; Dept. of Food and Nutrition Sciences and School of Pharmaceutical Sciences, Univ. of Shizuoka, Japan

3   *Future Med Catalog.* and *British Medical Report.*

4   a)The Univ. of Wales, Aberystwyth, tested 81 varieties, of which 46 exceeded safety guidelines, some for minerals such as sodium and uranium (the latter rarely seen in tap water). b) Chester Public Health Lab. (UK), found 22 out of 51 with bacteria in excess of limits set for tap water. c) Suffolk Co, New York, tested 88 bottled waters and found a number of cancer-producing agents present in several. d) Another American team, in Pennsylvania, analysed 37 brands, of which 21 did not comply with US limits for exc175ess mineral contamination, and only one satisfied EEC and WHO limits in every particular.

5   Fowles, Prof Gerry, "Yeast and Chlorine", NGWBJ, *Winemaking Magazine.*

6   Densley, Barry, "The Problem with Poisonous Plastics", *Nexus New Times,* Nov. 1996.

CHAPTER 7

A - Z: HOW TO HELP SPECIFIC DISEASES
AND IMBALANCES WITH KOMBUCHA

NB: These recommendations are no substitute for medical supervision. For serious conditions always consult your health practitioner.

In this section we describe each disease or imbalance and give medical research references where we can. This is followed by information and advice using Kombucha in various forms that will assist healing. We have researched, or personally been given these recommendations through the Kombucha Tea Network UK because they have been effective. Where we can, we have also given medical research information and anecdotes.

Kombucha is a nutritious health food drink in itself. But, in addition, we have suggested other beneficial dietary advice and lifestyle changes.

KOMBUCHA RECOMMENDATIONS WILL TAKE VARIOUS FORMS OF APPLICATION:

- **Kombucha Tea - as a drink** (*See* "The Dosage", page 46)

- **Kombucha Tea - applied topically** on the skin using a pad of cotton wool soaked in Kombucha tea. Squeeze out excess and apply to the affected area. Repeat as necessary.

- **Kombucha Cream** - liquidize small pieces of the fungus in an electric blender and use on its own or add this to a base cream (*See* Chap.13, "Kombucha Recipes").

- **Kombucha Poultice** - use a whole fungus or cut a piece as required. Secure with a dressing (melolin is good), and cover with cling-film or plastic wrap, if necessary. Bandage and re-apply as directed.

- **Kombucha Compress** - use a clean absorbent piece of fabric folded into several thicknesses and soak in Kombucha Tea - hot for chronic pain and cool for acute. Wring out to remove excess liquid. Cover with cling-film if necessary. Apply a dressing or, for large areas, cover with an old towel and rest. Re-apply as directed. If using a Kombucha compress in the area of the eyes, dilute it 1:1 with water

- **Kombucha Bath (full)** - add 500-mls-1-litre/1-2 pints of Kombucha tea or 2 cups of Kombucha vinegar to the bath water just before entering.

- **Kombucha Bath (pelvic)** - add 200-mls/1-cup of Kombucha tea or 30-mls/2 tablespoons of Kombucha vinegar* per 2-litres/4-pints of warm water to a bowl big enough to cover your lower pelvis.

- **Kombucha Footbath** - add 200-mls/1-cup of Kombucha tea or 30-mls/2 tablespoons of Kombucha vinegar* to a bowl containing 2-litres/4-pints of warm water.

- **Kombucha Douche** - add 30-mls/2 tablespoons of Kombucha vinegar* to 1-litre/2-pints of warm water in a medium-sized bowl. Use a clean soft flannel or cotton wool pad to soak and bathe the affected area for several minutes. Repeat as necessary.

- **Kombucha Hair Rinse** - pour Kombucha tea over as a final rinse. For more serious hair and skin complaints wrap hair in a polythene bag. Leave for 1-3 hours before rinsing off with clean water.

☺**Kombucha Sponge** - use a spare Kombucha fungus as a final rub down in the bath or shower.

⚱ **Kombucha Steam Inhalation** - add 200-mls/1-cup of Kombucha tea or 60-mls/4 tablespoons of Kombucha vinegar* to 1-litre/2-pints boiling water in a bowl. Immediately cover head with a towel, hold over the bowl and inhale deeply through the nostrils. Do this for at least 5 minutes, topping up with boiling water and fresh Kombucha tea when cooled. (**NB**: do not go outside for at least 2 hours, as the bronchial tubes will be open and vulnerable).

⚱ **Kombucha Drops** - Dilute Kombucha tea 1:1 with water and use in a dropper bottle.

⚱ **Kombucha Nasal Spray** - Dilute Kombucha tea 1:1 and use in a small bottle spray.

* to make **Kombucha Vinegar** - *See* Chap. 13, "Kombucha Recipes"152.

NB: Take care with Kombucha in topical use: poultice, compress and hair rinse, as Kombucha liquid can stain clothes and linen if made with black tea. Kombucha made with green tea is not likely to stain.

OTHER abbreviations:

🛝 **Research**

✓ **What *is* beneficial to do**

✗ **What is *not* beneficial to do**

📄 **Information**

A **Anecdote**

These recommendations do not take the place of medical supervision. In cases of serious illness always consult your health practitioner.

ABSCESS (and **BOILS**)

Abscesses or boils are caused by an excessive amount of pus (staphylococcus bacteria) in a confined space. They are very painful, indicating toxicity in the body and poor immune functioning.

⚱ Drink Kombucha tea regularly to detoxify and improve body functions.

☺Apply a Kombucha poultice to abscess, using a small piece of culture with a dressing. Re-apply morning and evening. In addition, we recommend covering the abscess with a warm/hot Kombucha compress to reduce pain and inflammation, and applying the Kombucha poultice in between. If it is a dental abscess, compresses can be used until an orthodontist can be consulted

A The above method was used very successfully by a woman whose medical treatment from her doctor failed to help a painful abscess under her arm. So she decided to take things into her own hands, using a piece of Kombucha culture. By the next day the boil had drawn out and was well on the way to recovery and the pain had dramatically subsided.

ACNE
Is an inflammatory skin condition caused by the body attempting to excrete unwanted toxins. It is especially prevalent in teenagers, but can also affect some adults. Acne ranges from a few annoying pimples to lumps and spots which can become inflamed, leaving permanent scars and pitting of the skin. Areas most likely to be affected are the face, neck, chest, shoulders and back.

⚱ Drink Kombucha tea for detoxification.

⚱ Apply Kombucha tea topically. Its organic acids and pH components act as a mild antibiotic to cleanse and repair the skin. Can be applied as frequently as you like, but for a minimum of 5 times a day.

☺Use Kombucha Cream.

⚱ Enjoy soothing Kombucha baths.

☺Rub the skin with a Kombucha sponge after a bath or shower.

✗ Avoid foods rich in iodine, e.g. sea kelp and iodized salt.

✗ Avoid fast foods.

✓ Eat zinc-rich foods, e.g. shellfish, oysters, lobster, wheatgerm, wholegrains, cereals, peanuts, pecans, legumes, liver and turkey, or take a zinc supplement in moderation.

AGEING

There is well-documented evidence of people in Kargasok, Russia living to well over 100 years. These Russian centenarians attribute their longevity, not only to their outdoor work and living habits, but also to the yeast enzyme tea (Kargasok tea or Kombucha) which has been in their diet for many hundreds of years.

Degeneration takes place faster in people who lead an indoor sedentary life. A modern diet containing excessive amounts of refined carbohydrates and saturated fat coupled with an inactive lifestyle that uses up fewer calories results in a net surplus which the body preserves as fat. This excess places stress on a variety of organs, leads to poor circulation and toxic build-up and eventually reaches a point where cells can no longer subdivide and deterioration begins.

We all need a steady stream of antioxidants in our bodies to oppose oxygenated molecules which damage cells and give rise to such diverse physiological processes as ageing, inflam-mation, drug-induced damage, toxic build-up, degenerative arthritis, alterations in immunity, cancer and cardiovascular disease, etc.

Kombucha has several main sources of antioxidants: methionine and vitamin C and enzymes. When the amino acid methionine, couples with pyridoxine (vit.B6), it forms a powerful antioxidant which provides protection from the toxic effects of smoking, alcohol and pollution.

Dr. E Arauner (1929) reached the following conclusion: "In summary one can say that the Kombucha mushroom or its extract has proven itself as excellently prophylactic against diabetes, but especially against ageing problems such as arteriosclerosis, high blood pressure with its consequences such as dizziness, gout, rheumatism, intestinal lassitude, haemorrhoids, tiredness and nervousness". He

reported that in Russia "the tea-mushroom has been in use for centuries by Asian people because of its surprising healing successes, being a most effective, natural home-remedy". Arauner added, "Not only professors, doctors and biologists have confirmed the surprising healing successes, but also those who have imbibed the mushroom-tea report: 'entirely excellent effects on the general body functions'".

Drink Kombucha tea as part of your daily regime for long life and good health!

✓ Eat foods with high concentrations of antioxidant activity - mostly found in plant foods such as: onions, lettuce, green vegetables, oranges, seafood, asparagus, avocado, cereals, spices, chili pepper, garlic (particularly good, as it has at least 15 different antioxidant chemicals).

✓ Exercise and fresh air are very important

AIDS

Acquired Immune Deficiency Syndrome is caused by a virus which affects the immune system and grossly depletes the T-lymphocytes (T-cells) by allowing opportunistic infections to take place. Depending on the general health and attitude of the sufferer, patterns of ill-health can include; a chronic continuation of glandular-type fever, swollen glands, night sweats, loss of weight and energy, herpes and Candida. Full blown AIDS can lead to the development of further serious symptoms.

Drink Kombucha tea as a nutritious health food drink, to strengthen the immune system and restore energy.

A Kombucha poultice or compress can be used successfully on scabs or skin lesions. Re-apply 2-3 times daily.

AIDS and HIV+ communities in the US report that components in Kombucha have shown positive results by inactivating viruses, assisting in weight gain and raising T-cell counts. Additionally and importantly it has empowered people.

▤ Seek help from a professional nutritionist for guidance on how to stimulate the thymus gland responsible for T-cell functioning. Nutrients which do this are arginine, vitamins A, C, E and B6 and the minerals selenium (especially), and magnesium - and how to clear the body of Candida (*See* page 78), which commonly affects people with AIDS. **NB**: Latest evidence suggests that zinc may stimulate the HIV virus.

ALCOHOLISM

Alcoholism is a disease like any other illness. It is a physical and emotional addiction which, in addition to seriously damaging the body, anaesthetises feelings, often bringing about shame, loneliness and even a dramatic change of personality in sufferers.

▯ Replace a drink of alcohol with a glass of Kombucha tea as often as possible, whenever you feel the need for a 'lift' or a 'kick'.

◒ Share a bottle of Kombucha with a friend.

▤ Kombucha has been shown to play an important role in alcohol recovery by reducing the craving for alcohol. The amount of alcohol present in Kombucha is no more than that contained in fresh fruit juice.

A One alcoholic man reported, "Kombucha tea reduces my craving for alcohol when I drink it all day". Another said, "It slows me down when I am on a binge". We even heard from someone who claimed, "It minimises a hangover when Kombucha is mixed with the booze" - which isn't quite what we're aiming for, but could form a significant part of the weaning off process!

✔ Be honest with yourself. If you can't go without a drink, recognise that you have a problem. Find an experienced counsellor to help you find the cause of the problem and go to AA (Alcoholics Anonymous) for support.

✔ Eat a fresh and nutritious diet, get lots of fresh air and befriend the natural world - the trees and earth can be healers too.

✔ Take plenty of honey which is a very good source of potassium and often deficient in alcoholics.

ALLERGIES

The term 'Allergy' is derived from two Greek words meaning 'altered reaction'. Individuals can suffer allergic reaction to, for example, house dust, dog or cat fur, food or chemicals. Symptoms include headache, migraine, rashes, asthma, vomiting, joint inflammation and lassitude.

Changes in western diet from whole and fresh, to a refined and processed one, with the use of food additives, herbicides and pesticides; in addition environment pollution in our day to day .living, slowly and surely diminishes the body's effectiveness for 'normal' functioning and immunity. This brings about food intolerances and allergic reactions for a growing number of people, and at an earlier age than before.

🕎 Unexplained attacks of joint pain is sometimes mistaken for rheumatoid arthritis. D. N Golding, a rheumatologist at Princess Alexandra Hospital in Harlow Essex, England, has documented what he calls "allergic synovitis", an inflammation in joint cavities that cause pain and swelling especially during bone movement. People most affected are those suffering from allergies and hayfever. The main food culprits are dairy foods and eggs. In a study back in 1943, it was found that 20% of patients who were 'allergic' had rheumatic attacks.

▯ Drink Kombucha tea as part or your daily health regime of detoxification and strengthening the body's immunity which can alleviate food intolerance and allergies.

▤ (*See* Case Study, p.116)

✖ Avoid stress and over-consumption of alcohol.

✖ Smoking impairs digestion and the body's health.

✖ The pill has a major influence on metabolism, which can affect food intolerances.

✓ Follow a food exclusion diet to determine the offending food(s) causing the allergy. This is best done under the supervision of a health or medical practitioner. Offending foods can include: grains - wheat, oats, rye and corn, dairy products, eggs, chicken, pork, sugar, chocolate, alcohol, citrus fruits, peanuts, yeast, colourings and preservatives.

✓ People who are deficient in certain vitamins and minerals (possibly iron, zinc or magnesium) mistake their poor state of health for a food intolerance. Make sure of an adequate balanced diet or consider good ('food state') nutritional supplements for 2-3 months to see if this helps. (*See* "Resource Section and Suppliers")

✓ Fresh air, sunlight, exercise and good sleep are of enormous value in creating a positive environment and attitude for the body to function at its optimum capacity.

ANAEMIA (IRON DEFICIENCY)

Anaemia only becomes significant if the body continues to lose blood at a rate faster than it can replace red cells, e.g. from heavy periods, bleeding piles or a failure to form sufficient haemoglobin because of deficient iron absorption. Iron comes from food and is stored for future use mainly in the liver, which is why animal liver is such a rich food source. At times of growth and during pregnancy iron can become depleted. Symptoms include pale ridged nails, cracked mouth, brittle hair, fatigue, weak appetite, and poor growth generally. There is usually a very obvious heartbeat on exertion.

Ʊ Drink Kombucha tea on a regular basis.

✘ Avoid tea and coffee as it will inhibit iron absorption.

✓ Foods rich in vitamin C help the absorption of iron from food, e.g: rosehips, apricots, bananas, cherries, blackcurrants, beetroot, potatoes, red kidney beans, watercress, black strap molasses, most green vegetables and liver.

ANAEMIA (PERNICIOUS)

This is usually, though not always, a disease of middle or old age. Some people suddenly begin to develop a sore tongue and cracked lips, a year or so later becoming pale and jaundiced, finally experiencing numbness or tingling in the limbs which can result in paralysis. Pernicious anaemia is related to the stomach whose peptic cells bind vitamin B12 and facilitate its absorption in the small intestine. Without it, this vitamin simply passes through. In some people in the 40-60 age range, the peptic cells of the stomach atrophy due to an imbalance in the auto-immune system. Orthodox treatment is to give vitamin B12 injections.

Ʊ Drink Kombucha tea (which contains vitamin B12) on a regular basis, to strengthen the immune system and improve functioning of the gastro-intestinal tract to ensure absorption.

A Kombucha helped a person with pernicious anaemia who was still experiencing numbness in the feet even after many years of having B12 injections from her doctor. After starting to drink Kombucha, feeling returned to the soles of her feet, first as a painful tingling. The sufferer gradually became able to feel the ground beneath her feet again and the improvement continued until normality was attained.

✓ Vegetarians, and vegans in particular, need to be aware of the importance of getting sufficient vitamin B12 in their diet. Sources other than meat and offal include oysters, onions, mushrooms, lettuce, milk, molasses, brewers yeast, fish, comfrey, eggs, bean sprouts, beer and stout; also in small amounts in spirulina, tempeh and miso.

ANGINA (PECTORIS)

Chest pain or angina is a symptom (not a disease) and a warning sign that the arteries are getting narrow (arteriosclerosis) or partially blocked so that oxygen and blood cannot flow easily. It can also result in heart spasms. Chest pain is linked to low blood levels of antioxidants (*See* AGEING). A susceptible person may experience angina after a heavy meal, excitement or exertion.

🕯 Dr. Mollenda (1928) discovered a new area in which Kombucha proved particularly helpful: "In the case of angina, especially where there is coating of the tonsils, the drink should not merely be used for gargling, which brings fast recovery, but for drinking also".

✓ Regular drinking of Kombucha tea (especially using green tea) will help to clear arteries and provide the body's regular need for antioxidants.

▤ (*See* Case Study, page 125)

✘ Stop smoking.

✓ Overweight people should reduce weight and enjoy gentle exercise.

✓ Eat plenty of foods rich in antioxidants: vegetables, fruits, oily fish, cereals, nuts, vegetable oils rich in vitamin E, and lots of garlic.

ANIMALS (*See* Chap. 14)

ARTERIOSCLEROSIS
This condition is a hardening of the arteries. It is caused by the arterial walls losing their elasticity and becoming blocked with plaque which is formed by cells, connective tissue, fats and calcium deposits, making the arteries narrow and affecting blood flow. A major concern is the possible abnormal clotting of blood which can cause a heart attack or stroke.

▤ (1927) Dr. Madaus revealed in "Biologic Healing Arts", that "The 'mushroom' has the ability to regenerate cellular walls and for this reason is particularly helpful in arteriosclerosis".

∪ Work up to a full regime, drinking Kombucha tea (use green tea, *See* Chap.6) to assist in dissolving artery deposits, creating elasticity in the cell membranes and improving circulation.

✘ Cut down on foods which contain fats and sugar.

✘ Stop smoking.

✓ Eat plenty of fish - particularly fatty fish containing omega-3 fatty acids such as mackerel and bass, or take fish oil capsules.

✓ Enjoy fresh fruit and vegetables.

✓ Fresh air and exercise is beneficial.

ARTHRITIS AND RHEUMATISM
There are many kinds of arthritis and rheumatism caused through inflammation, wear and tear, or by infections. The condition results in varying intensity of swelling, stiffness, pain and reduction of mobility. Conventional treatment is with anti-inflammatory drugs which reduces the pain and swelling, but doesn't deal with the problem. Arthritis is a condition caused by an accumulation of toxins in the body and sufferers usually have imbalanced liver functioning.

▤ (Hans Irion 1944) "Kombucha helps painful body-joints by transforming damaging deposits such as uric acid and cholesterol into easily soluble forms, thus removing them by excretion via the kidneys and intestines."

▤ "Glucuronic acid, one of the most significant organic acids found in Kombucha, and normally found in a healthy liver, is a most potent and effective detoxifying agent. Glucuronic acid is also beneficial when transformed into glucuronides and hyaluronic acid which affects the structures connected with collagen, cartilage and synovial fluid. A replacement of the deficient joint fluids and cartilage would reduce swelling and pain."

▤ It depends how far advanced the arthritic state is as to the degree of improvement gained with Kombucha, but most people find some improvement.

▤ Vitamin B3 (niacin) in Kombucha is also beneficial to arthritic sufferers, assisting improved blood flow to joints. Arthritis should be treated in combination with Kombucha and a change in diet.

▤ Prof.Dr.Wilhelm Henneberg (1926) recollects that "an unfailing remedy against joint rheumatism was made with this mushroom".

∪ Drink Kombucha tea to detoxify the body and strengthen the immune system.

☺Apply a poultice or a hot compress to the area of pain.

⎇ Take warm Kombucha baths.

☺Enjoy a Kombucha sponge rub down to help circulation.

A A great many arthritis sufferers, old and young, have reported a significant improvement when drinking Kombucha (including Alick & Mari).

✖ Avoid acid-rich foods such as rhubarb and citrus fruits, also foods from the deadly nightshade family (*solanacea* group) such as potatoes and tomatoes, as they have a negative affect on muscle enzymes.

✖ Avoid red meats, dairy foods, salt and sugar and drinks including tea, coffee and wine.

✔ Reduce weight if necessary and bring more gentle exercise into your life.

✔ Try magnatherapy (sometimes called biomagnetism) which involves the wearing of a magnet on the wrist or leg, or strapped to the back. The magnets stimulate the haemogloblin (red blood cells) which, as a consequence, are able to carry more oxygen around the body. Alick has been testing these for months and found that they reduced swelling and pain in the knuckles of both hands, and have significantly helped his hips. (*See* "Resource Section and Suppliers")

✔ Aid sleep with chamomile herb tea or valerian in the short term.

ASTHMA
This is characterised by recurrent attacks of wheezing, coughing and gasping caused by muscle spasms in the lungs and air passages constricting air flow. It can develop due to pollution, irritants, emotional upset, lifestyle and diet and can range from mild to life-threatening.

🕮 In a study in 1987, the physician and biologist Dr. Reinhold Wiesner published his results on a study testing the effects of Kombucha compared with the drug Interferon, which is sometimes used in cases of asthma (also kidney and liver dysfunction, rheumatism, AIDS, MS etc.). Kombucha gained better results than Interferon - 203 compared to 183.

🍶 Kombucha inhalations can be extremely beneficial

Ṳ Drink Kombucha tea

A It has been reported that; "Mucous cleared much more easily from the lungs when on a regime of Kombucha therapy and as a consequence my chest felt much more open. In addition, I had much more energy in the whole body".

🗐 (*See* Case Studies , pp.116, 127, 128)

✖ Definitely don't smoke!

✖ Avoid milk and mucous-forming foods, such as dairy, bread and potatoes. Coca Cola drinks have been known to bring on attacks. Also avoid food containing MSG (monosodium glutamate).

✔ Address the emotional situations in life that bring on attacks.

✔ Drink up to three cups of good (real) coffee per day. Research has shown that coffee has a broncho-dilating effect and relaxes the muscles surrounding the bronchial tubes.

✔ Hot pungent foods like chili, peppers, spicy mustard, garlic and onions make breathing easier for asthmatics by opening up air passages. They also have anti-inflammatory properties

ATHLETE'S FOOT
This is a fungal infection that lives on dead skin cells of the feet between the toes and thrives in dampness.

Ṳ Drink Kombucha tea three times a day.

🍶 In the evening enjoy a Kombucha foot-bath.

🍶 Use Kombucha tea topically whenever it is needed but especially first thing in the morning and last thing at night.

☺Use a Kombucha poultice or compress between the toes taped in place, and wear an old pair of clean socks made from a natural fibre.

☺Apply Kombucha cream alternately with topical use of Kombucha tea to help replenish and heal the dry skin.

A A supportive husband decided to drink Kombucha to keep his wife company when she started taking it for her CFS

(Chronic Fatigue Syndrome). He was amazed and delighted that his athletes foot problem, which he'd had throughout their married life, also began to clear up. Absolutely everything else in the past had failed, including all the preparations his medical practitioner had given him. He attributed his recovery to drinking Kombucha three times per day.

A My own personal experience (Mari) is that I developed raging athlete's foot for the first time in my life during a particularly stressful time. On first diagnosis I used only proprietary creams and powders from the chemists, as we were off on holiday and I had decided to have a break from Kombucha! There was no improvement at all to the hot, itchy and extremely painful symptoms (including skin falling off my toes). On our return home I threw everything away and decided that Kombucha was the answer. I drank Kombucha tea three times a day, used it topically during the day, and at night applied a poultice. Immediately there was an improvement, and within two weeks it had virtually gone and been replaced by new, healthy skin. I have had one more minor bout again during stress and it has been relieved instantly by using Kombucha tea and Kombucha cream. The moral of this story is *avoid stress* - and carry a Kombucha bottle with you at all times!

✗ Avoid walking barefoot in public areas like swimming pools.

✓ Follow general advice for Candida (*See* page 78).

✓ Allow fresh air to the feet, so wear sandals as much as possible. In cooler weather wear only natural fibre socks and footwear.

BLADDER INFECTIONS

Forming part of the urinary tract, the bladder is a hollow organ into which urine is constantly being drained from the kidneys. The bladder expands and contracts as urine is collected and released.

Urinary tract or bladder infections are usually caused by common Escherichia Coli (not E.Coli 157, infamous for food poison-

ing!) bacteria entering the upper urinary tract after travelling upwards via the urethra. Women are more often affected than men because the female urethra is shorter, straighter and relatively wider than the male's.

U Drinking Kombucha tea is of enormous benefit because of its detoxification and elimination properties, assisting better kidney functioning. It also contains antiseptic properties which help disinfect and cleanse bacteria from the system.

∩ Use a Kombucha douche to keep the genitals clean and to reduce the risk of further infection.

∩ Regular warm Kombucha baths - full and pelvic - are very beneficial.

✓ Add ½-pint/300mls (US: 1¼ cups) cranberry juice to 1-litre/2-pints (US: 5-cups) fermenting Kombucha two days before the end of fermentation. This not only makes a delicious drink, but also enhances the therapeutic properties of the cranberries.

🜪 Drinking cranberry juice is a centuries-old remedy for recurring bladder infections. In 1984 Prof. Anthony Sobota, a microbiologist in Ohio, discovered the cranberry compounds that block infectious bacteria from clinging to cell linings of the urinary tract. In 1991 these findings were confirmed by Israeli scientists at the Weizmann Institute of Science. For recurring urinary tract infections drink at least 8-oz/225-mls (US: 1-cup) cranberry juice per day. Also try eating blueberries as they have similar properties.

✗ Avoid caffeine, chocolate and alcohol during an active infection.

✓ Drink lots of fluids, at least 1½-litres/3-pints (US: 7½ cups) a day which will dilute concentrations of bacteria in the urine and promote frequent urination.

NB: A 30% increase in water consumption for each person would improve general health by flushing out toxins from the body.

✓ Wear loose clothing made from natural fibres and go without underwear as much as possible.

BLADDER STONES

Bladder stones (calculus) consist mainly of crystals of calcium salts that have separated from the body fluids. Calculi can cause severe irritation and pain especially if they create a blockage. The tendency to form stones in the urinary tract can sometimes be avoided by drinking lots of fluids.

- A Czech scientist discovered that phosphate stones could be dissolved in the laboratory with glucuronic acid (present in Kombucha). Phosphate stones inserted in the bladders of rabbits dissolved over several weeks. The animals were given Kombucha 2-3 times daily and the stones gradually reduced in size, eventually being discharged through the bladder.
- Adopt drinking Kombucha tea as part of a regular health regime.
- ✓ Drink lots of water especially when first taking Kombucha - at least 1½ -litres/3-pints (US: 7½ cups) per day to aid the elimination of toxins via the kidneys.

BLOOD CIRCULATION

Blood, 9-pints/5-litres (US: 11¼ pints) in a man and 8-pints/4-litres (US: 10-pints) in a woman, circulates continuously through arteries, capillaries and veins, carrying oxygen to every organ and tissue in the body where it is used in energy-producing chemical processes.

Blood vessel diseases are among the leading killers of the industrialised world. Loss of circulation leads to hardening of the arteries and signs of this vascular disease may begin to appear as loss of hair, thinning and atrophy of the skin, a purple or blackening colour of the skin (usually the extremities), pain on exercise, shortness of breath, fatigue etc. Poor circulation also affects the brain causing loss of memory and confusion.

Interestingly, a German doctor commented that "all illness has the common factor of poor blood supply".

- A vigorous Kombucha sponge-down is stimulating and good for the circulation.
- Massage with Kombucha cream.
- Enjoy warm and relaxing Kombucha baths.
- Drink Kombucha tea to keep the blood cleansed and well oxygenated.
- **A** An elderly gentleman described how his black/blue hands changed to a more healthy colour and were no longer cold after taking Kombucha tea for a number of months.

BLOOD PRESSURE

The pressure of the blood depends on the strength of the pumping action of the heart and the resistance produced by the smaller blood vessels. The term commonly refers to high blood pressure (hypertension), and low blood pressure (hypotension). High blood pressure can be hereditary, or caused by a stressful lifestyle, obesity, clogged arteries and defective calcium metabolism. Persistent high blood pressure can endanger the brain, heart and kidneys.

(Refer to the health benefits of Kombucha in ARTERIOSCLEROSIS, page 75)

- Drink Kombucha tea to help balance blood pressure, whether high or low (*See* page 18 - on adaptogens)
- ✗ Reduce stress levels, look at work/lifestyle. If your high blood pressure is stress-related, take a look at the causes, seeking help if needed.
- ✗ Stop smoking and find other healthy ways for support during stress.
- ✓ Begin a programme that aids relaxation and encourages doing what you enjoy in life.

CANCER

- Kombucha can be extremely beneficial for cancer sufferers and there has been an enormous amount of research done in this area (*See* Chap.9, "Kombucha Therapy with Cancer") (*Also see* DIGESTION, page 84, *and* Case Study, page 122)

CANDIDA ALBICANS

Has now been recognised as an important major disease-producing micro-organism found in MS, C.F.S and cancer sufferers, to name a few. It is present in everyone, and only a healthy gut will keep Candida under control and prevent its fungal colonisation. Potential Candida sufferers are likely to have taken one or several of the following: antibiotics or antibiotic-fed meat, anti-inflammatory drugs, the contraceptive pill, or have been bottle-fed as babies. Symptoms include fatigue, thrush (vaginal/oral), cystitis, bloating, fungal infections, including athlete's foot (*See* page 76).

It is important to starve the Candida and destroy it.

▤ Since Kombucha is often called a 'mushroom' or 'fungus' and also because it is a yeast as well as a bacterial ferment many people (including naturopaths) throw up their hands in horror and advise their Candida patients not to drink Kombucha, without understanding or looking further into the research. Kombucha, is misnamed the 'Manchurian mushroom', because it is not a mushroom. Kombucha is a mixed culture, a symbiotic community of yeasts (candida friendly) and bacteria.

▟ In 1958 the Russian researcher Prof. F Barbanick reported that, "The tea fungus bacteria energetically suppresses the growth of all other microbes", and in 1959 another Russian researcher, I. N. Konovalow, substantiated this by saying, "The potent growth of the Tea Kwass (Kombucha tea) directly suppresses the colonisation and growth of other types of yeasts and bacteria".

▯ Drink Kombucha tea to help correct nutritional deficiencies, combat yeast infection, repopulate the bowel flora and to strengthen the immune system and cellular membranes. Improved liver function will also detoxify the body.

⌀ Have a Kombucha douche any time, but especially morning and evening, for vaginal itching (thrush).

⌀ A full or pelvic Kombucha bath will be beneficial.

✖ Avoid all sugar, alcohol, tea, coffee, refined foods, yeast and fermented foods (**NB**: Kombucha has a different kind of 'yeast' which is beneficial).

✔ Do a herbal Candida cleanse. Seek a professional herbalist/naturopath or get a good book on Candida to help you (*See* "Recommended Reading" and "Resource Section and Suppliers").

✔ Eat plenty of 'live' yogurt to encourage the acidophilus properties to repopulate the bowel flora.

CHEMOTHERAPY and (RADIOTHERAPY)

Chemotherapy is the intravenous use of chemicals in the treatment of infectious diseases and of cancer. The side-effects can include loss of hair and yellowing of the skin and eyes.

✔ Because of its liver-detoxifying capabilities, Kombucha is extremely beneficial during treatment with chemotherapy and can help the body enormously to cope with the massive assault of chemicals upon it through detoxification.

▯ Drink Kombucha tea starting with a very small dose and building up gradually to the full recommended amount (*See* Chap.6, "Your Questions Answered" - The Dosage, p.46). If chemotherapy is repeated at intervals, monitor your body closely and vary the amount of Kombucha tea you drink, reducing and increasing the dosage as necessary. Consult a trained health practitioner when beginning the treatment. (*See* "Kombucha for Prevention of Illness and its Uses with Cancer", page 106).

A Many people have reported remaining reasonably well while drinking Kombucha, often experiencing little or no hair loss during chemotherapy, compared with other similar patients, even when doctors had advised and expected them to be much worse.

A A gentleman who began drinking Kombucha tea told us that he had experienced relatively trouble-free chemotherapy and, on the 3rd day of his 6-day course, actually felt 'uplifted'.

✔ Have a positive attitude and find out as much as possible about your diagnosis and treatment. Read and ask questions - *it is your body*. Also seek a local support group, this helps enormously for you and the whole family.

✓ Seek out an experienced and qualified healer who can help with emotional and psychological and perhaps physical aspects of your illness.

✓ Look at the many ways in which you can make your diet healthier by eating as much live and fresh foods as possible and introducing 'food state' nutritional supplements (*See* "Resource Section and Suppliers"; also the Bristol Cancer Help Centre).

CHOLESTEROL

In atherosclerosis (meaning hard porridge!) the lining of the arteries is covered in fatty deposits that contain large amounts of cholesterol. This causes a narrowing of the arteries and a lack of blood flow to organs, often resulting in loss of efficiency or failure. A sudden termination of blood flow can result in a heart attack. Cholesterol has a significant relationship as a primary or secondary precondition to certain diseases. There are two types of cholesterol, one - HDL (high density lipoprotein) - is beneficial to arteries, and the other, LDL (low density lipoprotein) is dangerous. Some foods are higher than others in cholesterol and diet can play a significant role in lowering LDL and boosting HDL. What you eat and drink can have an enormous effect on slowing the progression of atherosclerosis and even help reverse existing artery clogging by shrinking the clumps of plaque on artery walls.

≜ Dr. Rudolph Sklenar reported in the periodical *Experiential Healing Science*, "The 'Tea Fungus' is an outstanding remedy, which is a powerful agent for detoxifying the human body since it dissolves micro-organisms and cholesterol".

∪ Drink Kombucha tea (using green tea, *see* Chapter 6, "Kombucha - Your Questions Answered", page 43), both as a preventative and a cure.

✖ Avoid saturated animal fat found in meat, poultry and dairy products and eat only a very moderate amount of cholesterol-rich foods, such as eggs and liver.

✓ Foods that lower harmful cholesterol are beans, oats, bran, garlic, onions, salmon, mackerel, olives.

CHRONIC FATIGUE SYNDROME - C.F.S. (M.E. - MYALGIC ENCEPHALO-MYELITIS)

Has been misunderstood mainly because it resembles other conditions and because there are few tests that can prove the diagnosis. The main symptoms are muscular pain and stiffness, depression and profound fatigue. Medical research has looked in two directions as to the cause - metabolic and viral. The infective process associated with a virus is likely to cause damage to the immune system, which leads to a malfunction of the body's metabolism.

≜ A professor of clinical ecology (allergist) in the USA believes that food allergies are responsible in approximately 60% of patients who attend his clinic suffering from CFS. When certain foods are avoided they recover. The three main foods causing a profound reaction are: wheat, milk and corn.

∪ It is important when drinking Kombucha tea for the first time to take small amounts and gradually build this up to the full recommended amount. Taking too much too soon can be a strain on an already weakened system. Make sure also that your Kombucha tea is well fermented, and that all the sugar has been converted. Use pH test strips to be sure.

▤ (*See* Case Studies, pp.115, 116, 120)

A Some people with CFS have reported a 'healing crisis' when first taking Kombucha, which can be frightening if you don't know what is happening. (*See* Chap.6, "Your Questions Answered"). One confident woman with CFS, who understood what was happening to her, explained that all her symptoms had returned when she first started taking Kombucha. She decided not to cut back to a smaller amount and just continued with the full recommended amount. She said; "I watched my symptoms fall away one by one as the days and weeks went by and I moved through into improved health".

✓ Adopt a Candida diet (*See* CANDIDA) and Herb cleanse (*See* "Resource Section and Suppliers")

CIRCULATION (*See* BLOOD CIRCULATION)

COLDS (*See* Chap.8, "First Aid with Kombucha")

COLD SORE (*See* HERPES SIMPLEX)

CONSTIPATION

Hippocrates said that "death sits in the bowels, and bad digestion is the root of all evil".

Constipation is caused by a sluggish response of the intestines and colon which results in dry compacted material accumulating, and infrequent passage of stools. This waste residue can remain sticking to the walls of the colon and hardening over time, some of which remains embedded. In the warm conditions, this produces toxicity which gets into the blood system reaching every part of the body, eventually resulting in disease. Constipation will also affect the liver, gall bladder and kidneys due to toxic build-up.

Constipation creates in a person a sense of dullness, lethargy, emotional and physical blockage with lack of brain clarity and memory loss. It is more likely to occur in people who consume a diet of processed foods containing very little roughage and/or over-use of drugs such as antibiotics. Constipation can also be caused by illness, dehydration, obstruction (tumour or ballooning) or the attempted avoidance of pain on defaecation due to piles, etc.

📖 Kombucha is a lactic acid-fortified health drink which provides an acid environment that promotes the growth of beneficial lactobacteria (bowel flora) essential for a healthy colon. This aids the assimilation of nutrients and enzymes into the bloodstream and controls the putrefactive bacteria. A healthy colon = a healthy body/mind.

📖 Prof. Wilhelm Henneberg wrote that "A beverage made by means of the Kombucha culture, called tea kvass in Russia, is reputed to be a means of combating all kinds of illness, especially constipation". Dr. Maxim Bing also said, "Constipation caused by a sluggish response of the intestines may also be treated by this remarkable fungus".

🗍 Drink Kombucha tea three times a day, especially first thing in the morning.

📖 Within a few days of drinking Kombucha tea, most people notice a change in the frequency of their bowel movements which indicates that a cleansing process has begun to take place.

✗ Avoid mucous-forming foods such as potatoes, bread, cheese, pasta and eggs that bind the colon.

✗ Avoid using laxatives as they can be harmful, cause diarrhoea and worsen constipation by dulling bowel nerves so that they cease to contract normally.

✓ Drink plenty of fluids throughout the day - $1^{1}/_{2}$-litres/ 3-pints (US: $7^{1}/_{2}$-cups) made up mostly of water and the recommended amount of Kombucha. Fluid intake will, as well as cleansing the body, help bring about easier bowel movements.

✓ Eat plenty of live yogurt and fibre-rich food including fruits, vegetables, prunes, figs, dates, wholemeal bread and cereals.

✓ Coffee (both caffeinated and decaffeinated) in moderation can act as a mild laxative, usually being most effective in the morning. Over-use, however, can cause over-dependence and a sluggish colon.

CRAMP

Is a muscular pain caused by the muscle contracting and going into spasm. It occurs usually after prolonged violent exercise, resulting in a build-up of lactic acid, a waste product of muscular activity. Frequent cramp may be a symptom of poor circulation or excessive sweating.

🗍 Drinking Kombucha Tea will assist improved circulation and body functions.

🛁 Enjoy a Kombucha bath at night before going to bed.

✗ Avoid too much salt in the diet.

✓ Replace water if you have done vigorous exercise or been in a hot environment (such as a sauna) and only replace salt at the next meal. Do not take salt tablets or high salt solutions as they cause water to remain in the stomach too long.

CROHN'S DISEASE
This can affect the small intestine and any part of the digestive tract, producing ulcers and inflammation leading to tangled loops of the bowel known as adhesions. Typical symptoms are pain on the lower right side of the abdomen, attacks of diarrhoea alternating with constipation, poor appetite and loss of weight. The causes may be due to viral infection, allergies, diet or could follow an hereditary pattern. The disease may resolve itself in a few weeks or run a chronic course that may lead to other complications, such as anaemia and obstruction.

🔥 A group of British physicians at Addenbrookes Hospital in Cambridge has been treating Crohn's disease successfully for years with diet, believing that nutrition is even more successful than typical medication.

🍶 Drink Kombucha tea to restore colon bowel flora, fight infection and as a nutritious food drink.

✖ Foods likely to induce symptoms are wheat, dairy products, cruciferous vegetables (broccoli, cabbage, Brussels sprouts, cauliflower), yeast, citrus fruits, tomatoes and eggs.

✖ Also avoid whole grains, nuts and seeds, unless sprouted.

✓ Enjoy a mild, nutritious diet.

✓ Drink plenty of water and herb teas, e.g. chamomile, fennel and peppermint.

CUTS
(*See* Chap. 8, "First Aid with Kombucha")

CYSTITIS
This painful bacterial bladder infection can occur in many forms, acute or chronic. Symptoms may be extremely troublesome or mild. Generally there is the urge to pass urine frequently, even when the bladder is empty, accompanied by a burning sensa-

tion. This is a complaint common to many women, probably due to the shorter female urethra and its close proximity to the rectum where there is a greater risk of infection. Men can also suffer from cystitis. (*See* BLADDER INFECTION).

DANDRUFF
This is the common name for seborrhoea of the scalp, in which small flakes of dead skin form in the hair. It is caused by a disorder of the glands that secrete oil (sebum). There may also be a slight fungal infection, so check out Candida symptoms also (*See* CANDIDA).

🍶 Drink Kombucha tea.

🍶 Wash the hair at least twice a week and use a Kombucha hair rinse. Those with very short or no hair should rub the Kombucha tea into the scalp. Can be used for cradle cap, but dilute with water 1:1.

✖ Cut out tea, coffee, sugar and all processed foods.

✓ Follow a fresh wholefood diet.

DERMATITIS
The health of the skin is dependent on the nutrients it receives from the blood vessels in the underlying tissues, but it is also susceptible to outside influences and contact with toxic substances. Dermatitis is a rash caused by contamination of the skin by irritants such as bleach, washing powders, dyes, cement etc., if protection is not used. One example is ammonia in urine, which causes nappy rash. In normal medical treatment, much emphasis is placed on creams and ointments to localised areas, but it is also crucial to correct nutritional deficiencies and body functioning to get to the root of the problem.

🍶 Use Kombucha tea topically, either full strength or, for delicate skins, diluted 1:1 with water.

🍶 Rinse hands in Kombucha tea or vinegar immediately after you have been in contact with an irritant.

☺ Use Kombucha cream or a compress on the affected area.

☐ Drink Kombucha tea to correct nutritional deficiencies and body functions.

✘ Avoid skin contact with caustic substances.

✔ If you have generally poor skin, eat a good basic diet, making sure that you have a good supply of essential vitamins and minerals.

✔ Take 1 dessertspoon of cold-pressed linseed oil daily.

DETOXIFICATION

The body builds up varying amounts of toxins that can impair normal functioning, causing the liver and kidneys to become overloaded and perform less effectively, leading to disease. Toxins are removed from the body through a number of substances, the most effective of which is glucuronic acid (naturally produced by the liver) which binds up poisons and toxins, flushing them out of the body through the kidneys.

▤ Glucuronic acid is one of the major organic acids identified in Kombucha which provides an additional supply to the liver when its normal function has been impaired, thereby assisting more efficient detoxification.

▤ Analysis of urine has shown that people who drink Kombucha on a regular basis will also excrete specific toxins such as heavy metals; lead, mercury, caesium and benzol that have built up internally, and as a result of pollution from the environment.

▤ Author unknown: "One of the main reasons why Kombucha seems to be efficacious against such a wide spectrum of diseases is that it does not have any specific action on particular illnesses, but rather its systemic detoxification of the whole body through glucuronic acid has an overall beneficial effect that invigorates the entire person. When all the toxins have been successfully eliminated, the body is more able to heal itself".

▤ Günther Frank: "Can anyone be certain that their livers are healthy and functioning properly in these times of high pollution and toxicity, combined with contaminated nourishment and plenty

of stress? A healthy liver producing adequate glucuronic acid becomes critical when the environment contains excessive amounts of freely circulating toxic substances or when excessive amounts of endogenic metabolic toxins (from drugs and alcohol to junk foods) accumulate in the body".

☐ Drinking Kombucha tea is the first approach necessary in assisting the body's improved functioning. Begin gently by drinking small amounts and gradually build this up to the full recommended amount. This will prevent any discomfort in the detoxification process (*See* Chap.6, "Your Questions Answered" - The Dosage, page 46).

▤ (See Case Study, p. 128)

✘ Avoid: pollution, alcohol, drugs, antibiotics, cigarettes, sugar, processed foods and chemicalised water (includes tap, river-bathing and swimming pools).

✘ Ease up on stress.

✔ Enjoy fresh 'live' foods, preferably organically grown and drink plenty of good water.

✔ Exercise to your own ability and energy level, which will further improve body functioning and elimination.

DIABETES (MELLITUS)

Diabetes is the disease in which the body is unable to control the use of sugars as a source of energy. After a meal, blood glucose rises and insulin is released from the pancreas, helping the cells to take up the glucose and enabling the glucose level in the blood to return to normal. Young diabetics often lack insulin and older ones fail to respond to it normally. Thirst, passing of excess urine and weight loss are common symptoms of diabetes. There are two types of diabetics, insulin-dependent and non-insulin dependent whose symptoms can be managed with diet etc. Dietary advice to diabetics in the UK is given by the British Diabetic Association.

▤ 99.5% of the sugar that goes into producing Kombucha is inconsequential if it is made properly, as both the fructose and glucose produced are transformed into CO_2, organic acids and trace elements. When it is made correctly, Kombucha tea contains about the same amount of sugars as that in regular fruit juice. NB. Severe diabetic conditions should always have the supervision of a health professional when taking Kombucha.

U Drink Kombucha tea, making sure that the sugar has been converted in the brewing process by using pH test strips. (*See* "Resource Section and Suppliers")

▤ (*See* Case Studies, pp. 115, 125)

▤ Diabetics should monitor their blood sugar levels, and if necessary adjust insulin levels in consultation with their medical practitioner.

DIARRHOEA
Is the body's attempt to throw off an offending substance which has caused contamination through allergy, poisoning or infection. Long-term, diarrhoea will interfere with nourishment because bowel movements are speeded up, and food is passed through the intestines before proper absorption has taken place.

🕮 In an Omsk clinic, Russian trials into dysentery in infants treated with Kombucha showed that, after only a few days, diarrhoea had lessened and the children were gaining weight. After one week, no traces of dysentery were found in the faeces.

U Drink Kombucha tea to assist in elimination.

◔ Kombucha baths or douches are useful if there has been a bout of severe diarrhoea and the rectum is sore.

A Many people notice that their bowel movements regulate when taking Kombucha.

DIGESTION
The function of the digestive system is to break food down into simpler chemical molecules of fat, protein and carbohydrate so that they can be used by the body. The residue of undigested material is defecated.

Emotions such as sadness, anxiety, stress, love and grief can all have an affect on digestion.

▤ As a lactic acid ferment, Kombucha is known to rebuild the friendly intestinal flora, lactobacillus acidophilus, which is essential for healthy digestion, assimilation of food and metabolism.

A Tom Valentine:- *Search for Health* Magazine - "These 'God-given ferments' continue to serve human health far more effectively and economically than all the wonder drugs and complex compounds in the arsenal of modern science".

🕮 Dr. Sklenar noted during decades of medical practice; that "every chronic disease, including cancer is preceded by a general ailment of the organism, resulting mainly from metabolic malfunction. This triggers an increasing accumulation of waste material in the body and creates an ideal environment where a virus can develop - but not necessarily does". In this light, it is no surprise that the common saying, "No cancer patient has a healthy digestive tract" proves true.

🕮 Taken from a 1961 directory of 260 publications written by various doctors and researchers on Kombucha - Dr. L Mollenda (1928) wrote, "The Kombucha beverage proved itself effective, especially in troubles of the digestive organs"... "Even though the beverage is acid, it does not cause an acidic condition in the stomach; it noticeably eases and promotes digestion, even of difficult to digest foods" and "Kombucha is highly effective for digestive disorders due to its ability to balance and normalise the gastro-intestinal organs".

U Drink Kombucha tea to normalise pH levels in the stomach and assist healthy digestion and assimilation of food.

▤ (*See* Case Study, page 112)

A A gentleman told us that painkillers for severe back pain usually affected his stomach, but hadn't done so since he began drinking Kombucha.

A "It relieves my colitis and stomach cramps."

ECZEMA

This is a common condition which often begins in early childhood. The child who has a tendency towards allergy can become sensitized to any number of foods through the mother's breast milk. Children who were not breast-fed can become allergic to certain foods, mainly dairy products. Reaction can become chronic if not treated. Usually liver imbalance and/or poor immune functioning are major factors and certainly the case when sudden or constant stress leads to outbreaks of eczema in susceptible people, children and adults.

Ⓑ Scalp - use Kombucha tea as a hair rinse. The Kombucha may sting a little at first, but this will soon subside. Repeat daily if the problem is severe.

Ⓑ Use Kombucha tea topically, as an antiseptic to soothe and heal the skin; may be diluted 1:1 if necessary.

☺Use Kombucha Cream on affected area - carry this with you at all times in case of itching.

Ⓤ Drink Kombucha tea as a nutritional supplement to strengthen the immune system.

Ⓑ Kombucha baths will help enormously.

▤ (*See* Case Studies, pp. 116, 128)

A A female farming contractor in England who has had eczema for 20 years says that she has been 'cured' after drinking Kombucha tea.

✘ Children should avoid common allergens such as cows' milk, eggs, fish, cheese, additives and sugar. Adults should try a strict exclusion diet for 7-10 days.

✘ Look at the stress conditions in life and find a lasting improvement.

✔ If you have an eczema attack, look for certain triggers in foods.

✔ Correct diet deficiencies and try using a zinc supplement as many people with eczema have been found to be deficient in this mineral.

EMPHYSEMA

Is a chronic condition in which the air sacs of the lungs become enlarged. The condition can vary in degree of severity, with symptoms ranging from mild breathlessness on exertion to difficulty in breathing, wheezing, bluish skin and a chronic cough.

Ⓤ Drink Kombucha tea for improved body functions and to help clear mucous from the lungs.

✘ If you live in a polluted area, try to move to a healthier location.

✘ Giving up smoking - you may find that this alone arrests this disease.

✔ Massage and shiatsu are beneficial to release stagnancy and stiffness in the chest and lungs.

EYESIGHT

The most common defects of vision are short and long sight, astigmatism and deterioration through ageing.

A Many people have noticed an improvement in their eyesight using Kombucha therapy. They have included both those with impaired vision and those whose eyesight had been regarded as normal.

▤(*See* Case Study, page 112)

Ⓤ Drink Kombucha tea.

✔ If the eyes are relaxed the whole body is too - and relaxation of the whole body aids better eye functioning - try it, the two work hand in hand. (*See* Bates eye exercises and Meir Schneider ("Recommended Reading")

GALLSTONES

A gallstone is a small solid pebble-like mass (calculus) formed in the gall bladder. Many people have gallstones without the condition adversely affecting their health.

Gallstones may be associated with chronic inflammation of the gall bladder marked by nausea and can cause discomfort on the right side of the upper abdomen just under the ribs. There may be acute pain if a gallstone passes through the bile duct into the intestine. This is especially likely to occur after a meal rich in fat, which stimulates the flow of bile from the gall bladder.

🕯 Researchers at Bristol Royal Infirmary UK have shown that a diet providing the average amount of sucrose consumed in the UK produces an increased concentration of cholesterol in bile and therefore increased risk of gallstones.

🕯 Dr. S Hermann - "Glucuronic acid in Kombucha could dissolve gallstones".

🕯 Dr. Weisner - "Kombucha compared favourably with an Interferon product in gallstone treatment".

🗓 Drink Kombucha tea as a regular health regime.

✖ Avoid refined fats, carbohydrates foods and sugar and use olive oil in cooking.

✖ Lose excess weight slowly. Quick weight loss can bring on gallstones, so can fasting and skipping breakfast.

🗐 Gall bladder problems can be caused by frustration, suppression and anger.

✓ Eat lots of vegetables, especially legumes.

GOUT
Was once considered to be an affliction of the high-living, older, rich man, when in fact it can affect rich and poor alike. The average gout sufferer is a young man in his 20s-40s who usually develops intermittent pain at the base of the big toe. It is often confused as a strain or injury until it flares up. The problem is caused by uric crystals forming in the joints, kidneys and cartilage as a result of chemical processes in the body being upset. The preferred joint of the big toe is due to it being the lowest and coldest joint in the body, but other joints such as the knee and elbow may also be affected and develop excruciating pain when touched. If uric acid is formed very rapidly by the body, stones in the kidney may occur. (*See* KIDNEY STONES)

🗓 Drinking Kombucha tea has been well-documented by sufferers as an excellent remedy for gout throughout the centuries, due mainly to glucuronic acid's detoxifying properties, but also because of its action as a diuretic in flushing the kidneys.

✖ Avoiding rich foods such as red meat; game, liver and kidney and dairy products can be successful in preventing further attacks.

✖ Avoid excess salt intake and sodium-rich foods such as processed foods high in MSG (monosodium glutamate).

✓ Drink plenty of water, at least 1½-litres/ 3-pints (US: 7½ cups) per day to prevent uric concentrations building up.

HAEMORRHOIDS
A haemorrhoid is an enlarged vein in the wall of the ano-rectal canal which can bring extreme discomfort and pain, and may be accompanied by bleeding. Causes can be excessive straining due to constipation and excessive use of laxatives. Haemorrhoids can also develop during pregnancy when the foetus pushes against the abdominal organs.

☺Apply Kombucha tea topically or use Kombucha cream.

🧴 Before bed, apply a poultice or compress to the anal area, secured by the cheeks of the buttocks or tape.

🧴 Warm Kombucha baths, pelvic or full, will be extremely beneficial for the haemorrhoids themselves and also for the muscle encircling the anus.

🗓 Drink Kombucha tea to help alleviate the cause of the haemorrhoids such as constipation, gastro-intestinal problems, fluid imbalance, etc.

HAIR LOSS (ALOPECIA)
Hair loss is most noticeable on the scalp but can also occur on other parts of the body. Excessive hair loss can be caused by eczema, psoriasis, dermatitis, or nutrient deficiencies. Baldness in men is usually hereditary, women's hair may thin out too in older age or pregnancy. Sometimes hair loss can happen suddenly in an isolated patch (*Alopecia Areata*). Fortunately most cases recover spontaneously, though others can take months or even years. The cause is said to be unknown, but in the cases we have come

across, sustained stress would appear to be a major factor.

U Drink Kombucha tea.

⬯ To speed up the process of hair growth use a Kombucha hair rinse, or massage regularly into the scalp.

▤ (*See* Case Study, page 127)

A Some people have found their hair beginning to grow back while drinking Kombucha. It is often noticed as fine baby hair, very gradually getting longer and stronger. This has been reported even after decades of baldness.

✖ Avoid using 'the Pill' and other drugs which can also cause hair loss.

✔ Correct nutrient deficiencies, notably; iron, zinc, protein, and vitamins B and C. (Although zinc supplementation has had some degree of success with hair loss, it should be noted that in the long-term it should be supervised by your health practitioner)

HEADACHES (*See* Chap. 8, "First Aid with Kombucha")

HEART CONDITIONS
Many diseases affect the heart, and parts of the heart itself can become inflamed or diseased, possibly after another illness. Loss of flexibility in the arteries serving the heart (arteriosclerosis) or fatty deposits in these arteries (atherosclerosis) are causes of heart disease. Severe asthma, bronchitis or emphysema will also put strain on the heart.

In heart disease poor food and lifestyle can be major causes in the destructive processes that block and harden arteries. Conversely, good diet and lifestyle can contribute to the prevention of heart disease; keeping healthy blood circulating, ensuring it doesn't thicken or clot, and cleaning arteries, preventing cholesterol build-up.

U Drink Kombucha tea (made with green tea).

✖ Avoid saturated animal fats and polyunsaturated fats.

✖ Don't smoke.

✔ Take one junior aspirin a day as an anti-clotting agent (Dr. Campbell-Brown)

✔ Use olive oil in cooking.

✔ Maintain a healthy diet of fresh green vegetables, oranges, cereals, nuts, fatty fish, garlic, onions, ginger and hot peppers, and red wine (an anti-clotting agent, in moderation!)

✔ Tea drinking, especially green tea, thwarts blood clots and protects arteries. (NB: the beneficial properties of tea are even more enhanced in Kombucha)

✔ Always have breakfast, skipping it triples clot-forming potential.

HERPES SIMPLEX (COLD SORE)
Is a virus of the herpes family and attacks either the mouth and lips (HS1 or *Herpes Labialis*) or the genitalia (HS2 or *Herpes Genitalis*) producing a blister which ulcerates and crusts over. The first attack usually happens in childhood and subsequent attacks cause the virus to re-emerge from its dormant state, especially during times of stress, tiredness or exposure to sun and wind.

☚ According to Prof. Richard S Griffith, at Indiana Univ. School of Medicine, amino acids in certain foods can either stifle or encourage the growth of the herpes virus. Adding the amino acid arginine to the herpes virus in cell cultures made it grow rapidly, whereas adding the amino acid lysine halted the growth and spread of the virus.

At the first sign (the tell-tale 'tingle') do the following:

⬯ **Lips & mouth** - apply Kombucha tea topically using a small clean cotton wool pad or cotton bud. Do this frequently by carrying a small bottle of Kombucha tea with you.

⬯ **Genitals** - Kombucha douche frequently.

- have a Kombucha bath (full and/or pelvic) morning and evening.

- apply a Kombucha compress at night.

U Drink plenty of Kombucha tea for elimination and improved digestion, (in Chinese Medicine, herpes is connected to imbalanced stomach functioning).

✖ Avoid arginine-rich foods which can bring about an attack overnight. These include chocolate, nuts and gelatin. Eating foods high in arginine during an attack can exacerbate the condition.

✓ Eat lysine-rich foods such as; milk, soya beans, meat (including beef and pork), fruits, vegetables and bean sprouts. Edible seaweeds have been found to block herpes activity.

✓ Get plenty of rest.

HOT FLUSHES (*See* MENOPAUSE)

HIVES (*URTICARIA*)
Is a chronic allergic reaction which forms a reddish rash or circular weals that itch and burn on the surface of the skin. In some cases they last for only an hour or two, while in others they remain for several days.

U Drink Kombucha tea.

◊ Kombucha baths will be excellent.

◊ Use Kombucha tea topically or cream to calm and assist healing.

INGROWING TOE NAIL
Often the big toenail is the culprit as it has a tendency to curve into the flesh at the sides. It is usually extremely painful and has to be dealt with on a regular basis by a chiropodist to prevent inflammation and risk of infection.

A We were told of a successful treatment - a small piece of Kombucha culture was applied to the nail and replaced twice daily with a fresh piece. The inflammation quickly subsided, bringing relief. After one week the nail had softened and could be eased up and away from the toe using a cotton wool bud, gradually releasing the pressure and changing the direction of the nail. This is obviously a gradual and delicate operation and should only be undertaken if you feel confident and able to do so.

◊ A Kombucha footbath will assist the process also.

✖ Avoid ill-fitting shoes.

IMPETIGO
Is a contagious infection caused chiefly by staphylococci and sometimes streptococci bacteria. It can occur at any age, but is most common in babies and children. It generally appears on the face, hands and limbs, beginning with redness of the skin, and developing into blisters which break open to leave yellowish crusty sores that easily spread if picked.

▤ The antibacterial agents in Kombucha will stop the spread of the infection as well as easing the itching and preventing scars.

◊ Gently remove the crusts with a pad of cotton wool and incinerate or put in a plastic bag and trash. Apply Kombucha liquid and repeat at frequent intervals with clean cotton wool.

◊ Apply a Kombucha compress or poultice and replenish every 2-3 hours.

INJURIES AND DISABILITIES - (OLD AND NEW)
We wanted to include these anecdotes that were sent us to show the benefits that can be gained from Kombucha on a wide range of disorders, including injuries and disabilities that happened years ago. The people concerned had resigned themselves to living with the discomfort and pain for the rest of their lives, with the prospect of their condition worsening.

A A married couple both found that taking Kombucha tea helped them with old injuries. The wife experienced relief from pain in an old knee injury caused by a riding accident in childhood. The husband found the pain in an area of two crushed discs in his back eased.

A A gentleman told us how he had had an accident 40 years previously which had left him with a painful left instep and a permanently swollen ankle. After several months of drinking Kombucha he reported a huge improvement and was so surprised because he had stopped hoping for any after such a long time.

A A man who served for 18 years in the Indian Army was very fit until the onset of Spinalitus resulted in persistent pain between his shoulders and around his ribs. After a couple of weeks drinking Kombucha tea noticed the pain was almost gone and he was feeling and walking much better.

INSOMNIA
Is a problem that affects most of us at some time in our lives. The causes can vary from depression, worry or mental distress, to simply being uncomfortable or over-active. If insomnia is a persistent problem, it is important to find the cause.

U Most people find that drinking Kombucha tea noticeably improves their sleeping pattern, even if they take it mid-late evening. There are however, some of us who find taking Kombucha in the evening acts as a stimulant and keeps us awake. So, if you are one who comes alive late in the evening, we recommend you take your final drink of Kombucha much earlier on.

Relax before going to bed by enjoying a warm Kombucha bath.

✗ Don't eat too late and avoid stimulants like tea, coffee and chocolate.

✓ Magnesium and calcium supplements can help insomnia, as can B vitamins, but don't take them late in the evening.

IRRITABLE BOWEL SYNDROME
This is a common disorder of the lower bowel, where regular waves of peristalsis that cause faeces to move through the intestines, become uncoordinated. This creates a colic pain, diarrhoea or constipation, accompanied by flatulence and abdominal distention. It has been found recently that disturbances in the autonomic nervous system also develop in other organs such as the gall bladder, lungs and bladder, which shows that this condition is a multi-system disease. IBS seems to be more common in women than in men and especially those people who are of an anxious disposition, emotional or are depressed.

Food sensitivities and allergies are thought to be factors put forward by a group of British physicians. Gerard E Mullin, MD., an immunologist at the Johns Hopkins University school of Medicine says, "There is clear evidence that certain IBS patients do have allergic-type reactions and get better when they stop eating certain foods". Allergic reactions are not typical, and in fact are delayed and occur in the gut where there is an abnormal imbalance of bacteria. Candida may initiate damage to the bowel wall which permits unwanted microbes to enter.

(*See* ALLERGIES, p. 73 and CANDIDA, p. 78).

U Drink Kombucha tea to build up the body's own health: better organ functioning, immune system and defence mechanisms to help bring the body back into balance.

(*See* Case Study, page 124)

✗ Cut down on situations that cause stress. Try to be more 'centred' and balanced. If there is a flare-up take stock of what is happening to you in life and seek some quiet time at home to reconnect with yourself.

✗ It is advisable to look at certain foods and give up eating them for at least three weeks to see if it helps, these include; grains- mainly wheat and corn, dairy products, chocolate, tea, coffee, citrus fruits, potatoes and onions.

✓ Doctors now recommend a high fibre diet including bran or psyllium which can correct abnormal bowel patterns, and if diarrhoea is the main problem bran will usually help to solidify the stools. If there is a sensitivity or allergy to wheat then replace bran with soya or rice bran.

(*See* Case Study, p 112)

ITCHING (PRURITIS)
Itching results from damage to tiny nerve endings in the skin. Moderate itching may be due to dry skin allergies or insect bites. More severe cases may be caused by infectious diseases in which a rash occurs, such

as chickenpox. Heat often accompanies itching, and scratching is instinctive, but may injure the skin and cause infection.

▨ Kombucha's antiseptic properties will disinfect and prevent skin infection.

Ʊ Drink Kombucha tea to strengthen the body's immunity.

◌ Apply Kombucha tea topically or use Kombucha cream.

◌ Soak in a Kombucha bath.

◌ Apply as a Kombucha compress or poutice to the affected area as often as necessary. For rectal itching, leave in place between cheeks or use tape to secure, (beware sitting down - you could leave a wet patch!).

A A boy of 15 from the Netherlands had a chronic skin complaint which lasted 4 years. The itching he experienced began in his arms and was worse at night. He scratched until his arms bled and finally was given penicillin for the infection that followed. Hospital specialists thought that the itching was caused by intestinal bacteria and more medicine was given without bringing about any relief. His mother started him on Kombucha therapy and, after only one week, the itching had gone. After 6 months the scars were hardly visible.

✘ Foods such as nuts, caffeine and chocolate have been found to cause itching and it's worth eliminating them from your diet for a few weeks to see if that helps.

KIDNEYS

The kidneys are a double organ lying high at the back of the abdomen on either side of the spine. Their main functions are to monitor and maintain a constant internal water, mineral and acid/alkali balance and to filter and eliminate waste material from the blood, passing it out of the body via the bladder as urine. The kidneys also control blood pressure. When the kidneys are not functioning properly they are unable to secrete urine and the three main constituents of blood - water, salt and urea - build up in the body c ausing oedema, hypertension

and uremia. Excess urea is extremely toxic to the body.

Ʊ Drinking Kombucha tea is very effective in promoting healthy kidney functioning. It acts as a diuretic, helps correct the pH imbalance and, through its glucuronic acid content, plays an important role in detoxification.

▨ (*See* Case Study, page 121)

▨ Theophylline in tea makes it a very beneficial diuretic, so Kombucha Tea is doubly effective.

✘ Avoid over-tiredness, stress and anxiety. The kidneys show stress first in the body.

✔ Foods beneficial for the kidneys are celery, coriander, cumin, garlic, chicory, juniper berries, nutmeg, lemon, licorice, garlic, onion, parsley, peppermint and aduki beans.

KIDNEY STONES

Are a small mass of solid matter composed mainly of calcium oxalate, or uric acid and the amino acid cystine. Stones may form in any condition in which the concentration of calcium in the blood is raised, in kidney infection and other diseases. Normally the body controls the pH level of urine, but with a poor immune system and an overload of contributing particles suspended in the liquid, stones can easily be formed. Small particles may be passed in the urine without your even knowing, but larger stones give rise to referred pain which radiates down into the groin, thighs and to the tip of the penis in men. One person in two passes the small kidney stones, which can be very painful. Alternatively, they can be treated surgically. Diet and fluid intake play a major part in treatment.

☙ Water as Medicine! Dr.Stanley Goldfarb, professor of medicine in the USA, actually writes this prescription for people with recurring kidney stones, "Drink two 225mls/8floz (US: 1-cup) glasses of water every 4 hours in addition to other fluids normally taken throughout the day". This sound advice ensures a constant flushing of the system and will dilute concentrations of minerals that can crystallize into stones.

✓ Drink Kombucha tea for healthy kidney functioning; to prevent stones forming and for the elimination of toxic compounds.

A A 60-year-old patient suffering from gout reportedly had his high levels of uric acid reduced and normal kidney function restored after drinking Kombucha. His kidneys had not worked properly since childhood (Dr. Harnisch - in Tietze)

✓ Drink lots of water - as Dr. Goldfarb recommends!

✗ Avoid foods rich in oxalic acid such as rhubarb, spinach and peanuts.

✗ Avoid animal fats, dairy products and a high meat protein diet as they will interfere with oxalate absorption. People who form stones easily often have a high level of urates in their urine.

✗ Cut down on salt by at least half or remove from meals altogether. Also avoid high-sodium contents in processed foods, bacon and other cured meats.

✓ A vegetarian diet is wise. In Britain it has been found that vegetarians have only one third the frequency of kidney stones compared to meat-eaters.

LESIONS (*See* AIDS AND SORES)

LIVER (*See* DETOXIFICATION)

ME (*See* CHRONIC FATIGUE SYNDROME)

MEDICATION SIDE EFFECTS (*See* Case Study, page 128)

MENOPAUSE
When women enter menopause they can suffer side effects such as hot flushes and mood swings due to a reduction in oestrogen in their bodies. This reduction may also increase the risk of heart disease and osteoporosis (*See* page 93).

✓ Drink Kombucha tea to ease hot flushes.

✗ Avoid hot fluids as they are surprisingly also triggers for hot flushes.

✓ A glass of alcohol every other day is reported to alleviate menopausal problems. (N.B. It probably isn't the actual alcohol itself that is beneficial, but the oestrogenic activity from natural hormones in grains and hops that do good!)

✓ Eat calcium-rich foods, including an extra serving of greens per day.

✓ Soya beans and their derivatives e.g.; soya flour, tofu, tempeh and soya milk can stimulate oestrogen.

🔖 Dr. Forrest Nielson of the US Dept. of Agriculture found in studies that eating foods rich in the mineral boron boosts oestrogen levels to a "stunning level - as much as taking HRT (Hormone Replacement Therapy)". High levels of boron are found in fruit, especially apples, pears, grapes, raisins, peaches and grapes; in legumes, especially soya beans, in nuts including hazelnuts, almonds and peanuts and also in honey.

MIGRAINE
Susceptibility runs in families, but the term specifically indicates a headache caused by alteration of the size of blood vessels in the brain. This can come about due to stress, hormonal change, the contraceptive pill and consumption of certain foods. The attacks usually start on one side of the head and may include distorted vision, flashing or coloured zig-zag lights and difficulty in focusing. Later symptoms are the characteristic throbbing and bursting sensations in the head which can last for hours. If the attack is severe it can include numbness, tingling and be accompanied by nausea and vomiting.

✓ A regime of Kombucha therapy can be effective in the long term if the cause is toxicity, allergies or hormonal imbalance.

🍶 Apply a *cold* Kombucha compress to the forehead and temples for relief, and change frequently as it warms up.

🍶 A *warm* Kombucha compress applied to the back of the neck, helps to open blood vessels to the brain and will help ease the pain.

✱ Avoid the trigger foods if you are susceptible until the body comes back into balance: - caffeine (cut back gradually), chocolate, cheese, yogurt and soured cream, nuts, processed and cured meats, alcohol (especially red wine and champagne), MSG (monosodium glutamate), citrus fruits, pineapples and certain bread products. The most common trigger with children is cow's milk.

✓ Ginger has been used for centuries in some cultures to treat headaches and nausea. Like aspirin, and some automigraine drugs, it stimulates prostaglandins that help control inflammatory responses and pain.

⚖ Successful research trials showed - at the first sign of visual disturbances take 500-600mg (¹⁄₃ teaspoon) powdered ginger mixed with water, and repeat 1 dose per day over the next 3-4 days. Use fresh ginger regularly as part of a daily diet.

✓ Eating oily fish such as salmon, tuna, mackerel and sardines, and fish oil capsules can cut the number of migraine attacks by half and also lessen their severity.

✓ Restricted blood supply to the brain often accompanies migraine. Apply a hot/warm compress to the back of the neck to help increase blood flow to the head.

MULTIPLE SCLEROSIS
Is a disease in which nerve linings scattered in small areas of the brain and the spinal cord are attacked. In severe cases the nerves involved cease to function. Attacks happen mostly in young adults who may suddenly develop a variety of symptoms including numbness, pins and needles, weakness, blurred vision or impaired eyesight, difficulty in walking and dexterity. In typical form there are periods of attack and reprieve, with recovery in between and slow deterioration.

▤ Bob Banham's personal experience is an inspiration (*See* Case Study, page 112)

⛆ Drink Kombucha tea. (*See* Chapter 6, "Kombucha - Your Questions Answered" - The Dosage, page 46)

▤ Bob Banham has informed us that from the hundreds of people with Multiple Sclerosis whom he and his wife Nicola have supplied with a Kombucha culture through The Kombucha Network, he knows of *no-one* who has *not* gained some improvement in their health.

A From *Search for Health Magazine* USA - A woman in the Netherlands had suffered from multiple sclerosis since 1982 and began drinking Kombucha in 1989. At the time. she could only walk a few metres out of the house using two canes and her condition was worsening. She said that she experienced the detoxifying effects of Kombucha on the body with good results, and was able to go out for longer periods of 20 minutes without canes and didn't feel the extreme tiredness. A medical check-up in 1992 was positive, which resulted in her being able to hold a full driver's licence again and she has plans to try a little skiing.

NAIL INFECTIONS - (FUNGAL)
Can occur in gardeners, when strands of fungi lodge in cracks, discolouring the nail, pervading the keratin and separating it from its bed. A similar fungal disorder affects those people who have their hands in water frequently, causing inflammation of the cuticle, which becomes red and soggy.

A Dr. Campbell-Brown noted personally that after taking Kombucha for a few weeks, there was a marked increase and strength in the growth of his fingernails and found similar improvements in several of his patients.

◯ Try finger baths, holding the tips of the fingers immersed in Kombucha for up to five minutes. Repeat morning and evening.

☺When possible, but especially at night, apply small pieces of culture as a poultice to the fingernails and tape. Replace every 6 hours as the culture dries out.

NERVOUS DISORDERS
B vitamins are active in providing the body with energy all day and are important for normal functioning of the nervous system.

🗐 Kombucha produces most of the B complex vitamins: B1, B2, B3, B6 and B12, Thiamine (B1), Riboflavin (B2), Pyridoxine (B6), and especially Cycanocobalamin (B12) which are all water-soluble nutrients that the body needs to replace daily. Because Kombucha produces these complex B vitamins naturally, they are more efficiently absorbed into the bloodstream.

🗑 Drink Kombucha tea.

🗐 (*See* Case Study, page 129)

🝰 In trials zinc food status supplements have been shown to improve mental health disorders.

A An 80-year-old woman wrote to us, saying that after 2-3 days drinking of Kombucha she had a 'peaceful feeling' and, when she went shopping, instead of panicking as usual she shopped with pleasure and even mowed the lawn which she hadn't done for years.

OEDEMA
Oedema is a fairly common problem where there is an abnormal accumulation of fluid in the body, in particular the feet and ankles, which is made worse by standing and hot weather. More generalised fluid retention may result in swelling of the fingers and puffiness around the eyes and in the face. Oedema is not a symptom, rather an indication of a disease or imbalance.

🗐 Most people notice an increase in urination when first drinking Kombucha tea due to the body detoxifying.

🗑 Drink Kombucha tea for its diuretic properties and for balancing the body's system.

🗐 (*See* Case Study, page 117)

✖ Avoid excess salt which retains water.

✖ Avoid refined carbohydrates such as sugar, honey and glucose which require a considerable amount of water to be metabolised.

OSTEOPOROSIS
Osteoporosis occurs mainly in women and is due to the decline in circulating oestrogens and hormone imbalance around the time of menopause. The bones become so weak that they easily fracture or crumble. Men who develop osteoporosis suffer a great reduction in their new bone formation.

🗑 Drink Kombucha tea for improved body functions and absorption. (tea is rich in manganese which is beneficial for bones, and will be enhanced in the Kombucha fermentation.)

🍶 Regular warm Kombucha baths will be beneficial.

A A man in Austria has reported having found great relief from drinking Kombucha. He was in a poor condition and couldn't walk properly. After a few months taking Kombucha tea he found that he was gradually getting stronger. This has continued to the point where he is now able to lead a normal life again, walking and exercising. He says enthusiastically that he will drink the tea forever.

✖ Avoid smoking.

✖ Caffeine is also thought to promote calcium excretion, so high coffee drinkers are more likely to suffer hip fractures. Keep intake to under three cups daily.

✓ Enjoy exercise to strengthen bones and stimulate the activity of osteoblasts, which continually build up new bone.

✓ To prevent bones from becoming weaker, eat a diet sufficient in vitamin D (fatty fish is an excellent source, eel is especially high). Milk and sunlight are other good sources.

✓ The mineral manganese is required for bone metabolism, so regularly eat or drink pineapple which is readily absorbed. Other good sources are beans, cereals, wheat, oatmeal, nuts, spinach and tea.

✓ Have a good diet of high-calcium foods especially when you are young to build up density in bones and after the age of 30 to retard bone loss and prevent fractures.

✓ Foods rich in calcium are kale, broccoli, turnip greens, figs, dairy products, yogurt, fish, beans (soya beans in particular); tofu, and soya products, (notably tofu). (NB: calcium absorbed from kale is better than that from milk).

🜂 Dr. Heaney from The National Osteoporosis Society in Somerset, UK recommends:

- 1,000-mgs calcium daily for everyone over 14-yrs old

- 1,200-mgs for pregnant and nursing women

- 1,500-mgs for pregnant, nursing teenagers and women of 45-years and over who are not on HRT.

📰 Women from Asian countries have very little osteoporosis, even though their diet is low in calcium-rich dairy foods, but they eat high quantities of soya bean products and green leafy vegetables. (*See* MENOPAUSE)

PILES (*See* HAEMORRHOIDS)

PRE-MENSTRUAL SYNDROME (PMS)
PMS has been defined by Dr. Katharina Dalton in London as; "The appearance of symptoms in the premenstruum and their disappearance in the postmenstruum!". More than 150 symptoms have been described, with most women suffering between 1-6 of these. They include anxiety, irritability, mood swings, weight gain, abdominal bloating, breast tenderness, headache, craving for sweets, increased appetite, fatigue, depression, clumsiness, forgetfulness, crying, insomnia, confusion, feelings of violence or even suicide (actually, most women identify with more than 6 on this list!). It is recognised that other conditions are aggravated premenstrually.

📰 Many people have found that their PMS symptoms have been alleviated through drinking Kombucha tea. This can be attributed mainly to Kombucha's ability to detoxify the liver when it is overloaded with oestrogen. High oestrogen levels are also associated with a lack of B complex vitamins which are needed by the liver to break down and inactivate the oestrogen.

🜊 Drink Kombucha tea as a detoxifying health food drink and as a beneficial source of vitamins, including most of the Bs. Take it regularly, but especially the 2 weeks prior to your period.

🜍 Have warm Kombucha baths before and during menstruation.

✖ Avoid caffeine; it affects some PMS. women significantly.

✖ Reduce stress, and avoid making major decisions 1 week prior to menstruation.

✓ Eat calcium foods and have toast for breakfast. Research has shown that insufficient calcium and magnesium play a significant role in increased PMS symptoms.

✓ Carbohydrates relieve symptoms before and during a menstrual period, so don't deny your craving for sweet things, bread, pasta, potatoes, rice and cereals.

✓ Regular exercise is of proven value: walking, swimming, yoga, tai chi etc.

POST-OPERATIVE RECOVERY

A A gentleman who had his gall bladder removed complained of constant pain after the operation. When he started drinking Kombucha the pain eased.

PREGNANCY
(*See* Chapter 6, "Your Questions Answered" - Contra-indications, page 47)

PREVENTATIVE
Many people come to Kombucha because they have reached a stage where imbalance has developed into an illness. They are often despondent, or even desperate because conventional medicine has failed them. Through taking Kombucha tea, they discover the value of good health through self-help and a new interest in alternative approaches. But Kombucha can be of enormous benefit long before this stage. It can be used both to maintain health and to improve it in the future.. 'Prevention is better than cure'. - It make sense not to get ill in the first place!

U Enjoy Kombucha tea as a regular health regime.

A A family with three children of varying ages who take Kombucha say that they have all avoided the usual winter coughs and colds. The mother, a nurse, says she has more energy in her night duty work. She believes that Kombucha has certainly kept them all in better health - a claim shared by many other people who have contacted us.

✓ A herbalist reminded us of three simple rules for healthy eating: eat foods that are as whole, as local and as fresh as possible. You can add to this - and in season

✓ Always enjoy what you do, and don't do what you hate - it makes you ill!

✓ Take a look at exercise and relaxation.

PSORIASIS
Psoriasis is a mysterious inflammatory skin condition in which the rate of keratinisation of the epidermal cells is greatly speeded up. Instead of taking a month to reach the surface of the skin they accomplish this in only a few days. This causes the cells to stick together which results in the thickened skin having a silvery, scaly appearance which flakes off prematurely leaving a pink, patchy rash underneath. It is most commonly found on the arms, legs, elbows, knees and hairline, but can appear anywhere on the body. An over-toxic liver is associated with psoriasis.

U Drink Kombucha tea to help correct imbalances.

Apply Kombucha tea topically as often as required and/or use a compress.

Use Kombucha cream.

Take Kombucha baths regularly.

Many psoriasis sufferers taking Kombucha have reported substantial relief after years of discomfort and failed orthodox treatment.

✗ Avoid pro-inflammatory animal fats and omega-6 type vegetable oils such as sunflower, corn, safflower and margarines.

✓ Sunshine is beneficial, though care should be taken not to burn.

✓ Fish oil which contains anti-inflammatory properties helps, especially in salmon and mackerel.

RADIOTHERAPY (See CHEMOTHERAPY)

RASHES (See ITCHING)

RHEUMATISM (See ARTHRITIS and RHEUMATISM)

SCARS
A Dr. Campbell-Brown had a patient who developed M.S. at the age of 18 and fell frequently, damaging her limbs and leaving bad scarring. Twenty years ago she began taking Kombucha regularly. Since then, any skin injuries have healed without scarring. The patient is now 70yrs old and mobile, coping with other disturbances from M.S. but maintaining complete confidence in Kombucha. He believes her M.S. symptoms may have been worse if she hadn't been taking Kombucha.

Use Kombucha tea topically or Kombucha cream to promote healing of scars.

SERIOUS ILLNESS AND DISEASE
With serious conditions it is important to consult your doctor or medical practitioner. However, we believe that Kombucha therapy can also be beneficial at these times and, as a form of complementary medicine, can assist one's healing, in association with orthodox treatment. Kombucha tea may be taken in addition, and won't interfere with any other medication. Do discuss this with your practitioner.

We recently received a letter from a woman in Scotland who suggested including her experience in our book: After much uncertainty, she has had the disease PSITTACOSIS confirmed by her doctor. This condition is caused by a virus-like micro-organism, and is commonly transmitted to humans by certain birds (ducks, chickens, pigeons, parrots) which are infected. Eighteen months ago her son started her on Kombucha tea and she says "Although it hasn't cured the disease, I have felt *much* better on it, and it has helped to control and close the open wounds (on my skin)."

SHINGLES (HERPES ZOSTER)

Is a very painful condition where the herpes virus gets into nerve cells and causes circles of painful blisters on the skin. Sometimes known as 'the ring of roses from hell', shingles is caused by the same virus as chicken-pox. The pain, called post-viral neuralgia, can remain even after the blisters heal. Shingles mostly occurs in the elderly or when immune efficiency has declined, or where there has been a shock.

◌ Use Kombucha tea topically or use Kombucha cream.

◌ Apply a compress or poultice over the affected area.

◡ Drink Kombucha tea to support the healing process and for improved immune system functioning.

◌ Warm Kombucha baths will be very beneficial, but may smart at first.

✖ It is important not to give chocolate to someone who is elderly and susceptible to shingles, as this can bring on an attack.

(*See* HERPES SIMPLEX for other important dietary advice)

SINUSITIS

There are four sets of hollow cavities in the front of the skull called the paranasal sinuses. If one or more become inflamed or infected, it gives rise to a painful condition called sinusitis, where the nose is partially or completely stopped up with mucous. During a head cold, sinusitis can occur due to the connection with the infection in the nose. If the frontal sinuses are affected it can cause extreme headache. Sinusitis can also be caused by allergies, irritation from pollution or dry air, infected teeth and tonsils.

▤ Kombucha's antibiotic and antiseptic properties are extremely effective in cases of viral infection, inflammation and immune efficiency.

◌ Use Kombucha steam inhalations.

◌ Use a Kombucha nasal spray as often as required.

◡ Drink Kombucha tea for a deeper and lasting effect.

✖ Avoid common allergens such as dairy products, wheat, eggs, citrus and soya products and processed foods to see if this helps.

✖ Avoid all mucous-forming foods such as potatoes, pasta, milk, cream, etc.

✖ Sinus sufferers should avoid smoking or being in the proximity of smokers.

✓ Eat plenty of fruit and vegetables and drink mineral water, herb teas and vegetable juices.

✓ Hot, spicy foods including; hot chili peppers, curry spices, horseradish and garlic help break up congestion and flush the sinuses.

SKIN DISORDERS

Kombucha is very good for all skin conditions. In its propagation it grows a new layer - or skin. Nature is showing us one of its major healing properties. (*See* individual skin disorders; *see also* Case Studies, pp. 115, 123, 128)

SPONDYLITIS

May be due to injury or a disease such as arthritis or tuberculosis. It can be a persistent condition leading to inflammation, stiffness or deformation of spinal joints. Ankylosing Spondylitis affects mostly young men. Chronic conditions sometimes result in rigidity and curvature of the spine.

◡ Drink Kombucha tea as well as enjoying Kombucha baths

◌ Relax in warm Kombucha baths

◌ Apply a warm Kombucha compress to area of discomfort.

A Dr. Campbell-Brown's own personal experience is that within 2-3 days of drinking Kombucha tea, he experienced remission from his spondylitis onset and relief from severe neck pain.

✓ Regular gentle bodywork can be very beneficial.

STINGS (*See* "First Aid", p.100)

STROKE
Is damage to the brain as a result of blockage to an artery or bleeding from a ruptured artery in the brain. It can cause a sudden loss of consciousness and paralysis. Symptoms differ depending on which side of the brain is affected. The conditions mainly responsible for a stroke are hypertension (high blood pressure), arteriosclerosis, and valvular heart disease.

U Drink Kombucha tea (especially green tea) to clear arteries, promote good circulation, lower blood pressure and improve the body's general condition.

A A woman reported that after she had been taking Kombucha for 4½ months she was able to flatten her hand for the first time in 14 years since she'd had her stroke. She added that she was also walking better and that her circulation had improved.

✱ Avoid high-pressure jobs and long-term frustration.

✓ Follow a good diet (*See* ARTERIO-SCLEROSIS)

SUNBURN (*See* Chap. 8, "First Aid")

SWOLLEN ANKLES (*See* OEDEMA)

TENDINITIS AND BURSITIS
Tendinitis is the inflammation of a tendon, the band of tissue which anchors a muscle to the bone. Usually the condition involves tenosynovitis which is inflammation of the sheath surrounding the tendon. This condition affects the joints of the wrists and knees and is usually caused by repetitive movements in people who either play sports such as golf or tennis, or are in occupations like carpentry and the building trade. A thickening of calcium salts can develop in tendons, particularly around the shoulder joint (Frozen shoulder).
Bursitis is the painful inflammation of a bursa which is an accumulation of an abnormal amount of fluid, leading to the bur-

sal sac becoming swollen. Bursitis over the knee, otherwise known as 'housemaid's knee', results from the joint having been subjected to too much pressure and strain. Office workers may get bursitis of the elbow.

▤ Kombucha is extremely beneficial in improving the elasticity of tendons and ligaments and strengthening muscles. It also helps in clearing offending deposits from the joints. As well as helping in detoxification, glucuronic acid in Kombucha is used in the body to build important polysaccharides such as hyaluronic acid, which is vital for connective tissue, and chondroitin sulphate acid, the basic substance found in cartilage.

🍶 Apply a cold Kombucha compress or poultice to the affected joint. Re-apply morning and evening.

U Drink Kombucha tea to aid repair and restore normal functioning to the damaged tendon.

🍶 Warm Kombucha baths would be helpful.

A A person told us of his "great delight in having long-term pain relieved in an elbow. After drinking Kombucha tea for several months, it has very gradually and steadily improved".

A A workman who suffered for many years from bursitis in his shoulders, caused by repetitive movements involved in lifting, had his life considerably improved. After a few months drinking Kombucha he said the chronic pain had all but vanished and movement was almost back to normal.

✓ Ease up on repetitive pressure on the affected joint by being more aware of how you actually use it. Strain on the body can be caused by tension in everyday actions. Relaxation helps as well as re-learning how to use the body naturally (yoga, tai chi, shiatsu, the Feldenkrais method and the Alexander Technique are especially recommended).

THRUSH (*See* CANDIDA ALBICANS)

THYROID GLAND

Under the influence of the pituitary, the thyroid gland is at the base of the neck on both sides of the windpipe below the larynx, which can become enlarged (goitre). It produces the hormone thyroxine which regulates the speed of chemical reactions in the body (metabolism) and contains iodine which is a trace element and is provided in the diet.

The thyroid is susceptible to attack by anti-bodies (autoimmune disease) and may lead to under- or over-production of thyroxine. Inadequate production is called *Hypothyroidism* which can affect the skin, giving it a puffy, yellow, coarse appearance and can arise in some women of menopause age where the effect is a slowing down of bodily functions, leading to weakness and fatigue. *Hyperthyroidism* occurs when increasing quantities of thyroxine are produced causing enlargement of the eyes. Usually most frequently seen in young women where an increasing amount of energy is being metabolised, who have an enlarged appetite but accompanied by an unusual amount of weight loss. They may also suffer from high blood pressure, diarrhoea, scanty periods and inflamed and gritty eyes. Both under- and over-activity of the thyroid gland can result in low blood sugar (hypoglycemia)

U Drink Kombucha tea to help regulate and balance the metabolism and strengthen the immune system.

▤ (*See* Case Study, page 117)

✓ Evidence suggests that the recommended iodine intake of 100-mcg daily for adults and 150mcg for children, adolescents, pregnant and lactating women are not being met without the use of iodised salt (most table salt!). Foods which are rich in iodine include: fish - haddock, halibut, shrimps, oysters, clams and tuna; also seaweed, dairy produce, wholewheat bread, pork, lamb, lettuce, spinach, green peppers and raisins.

▤ Some experts are also concerned about the excess intake of iodine used in the dairy industry, in colourings and in dough conditioners, which can result in a skin condition similar to acne.

TONSILLITIS

Is inflammation of the tonsils and may be a symptom of other disorders. The ensuing infection can also affect other parts of the body. Throat conditions can also be connected to a lack of self-expression, not speaking up for oneself - repression.

▤ In Kombucha research trials in a clinic in Omsk, Russia, inflammation of the tonsils was treated with remarkable success. Patients used Kombucha to rinse their mouths ten times a day; the liquid being held in the mouth for fifteen minutes. (*Lebendsmittelrundschau* 1987)

U Drinking Kombucha tea warm can be comforting.

⌀ Gargle with Kombucha tea and/or rinse the mouth, holding the liquid for up to 15 minutes (as above) before spitting out.

ULCERATED LEGS

Although ulcers around the ankle are usually of varicose origin and can take many months to heal, they can also arise because of other conditions such as diabetes. African or West Indian people with sickle cell anemia are also prone to leg ulceration.

▤ Dr. Campbell-Brown has successfully treated leg ulcers which have been normally very difficult to heal. Below is the method of treatment that he used:

☺ Cover the ulcer with a piece of Kombucha culture, which is slightly bigger in size, as a poultice. Cover with a melolin dressing and cling film or plastic wrap to retain any liquid and apply a crepe bandage. Renew daily with a fresh piece of culture and a clean dressing. (*See* Case Studies, pp. 117, 123)

U Drink Kombucha tea to correct imbalances in the body's system.

VARICOSE VEINS

Are dilated and knotted blood vessels close to the surface of the skin and usually appearing in the leg. At intervals the valves that prevent the blood flowing backwards can become weak and unable to function properly. Varicose veins are more prevalent in women and may be caused by standing a lot. They can also occur during pregnancy. Varicose veins can cause inflammation, phlebitis and ulcers if neglected.

◌ Use a Kombucha compress over the painful area of the vein.

∪ Drink Kombucha tea to aid blood circulation and improve elasticity in the walls of the veins.

✓ Walking will help stimulate circulation in the legs. Rest the legs up between walks.

WARTS
Are small growths, usually benign (non-cancerous) and rooted into the skin. Ordinary warts, which tend to occur mainly on the face, hands and knees can be common in children and young people. A troublesome wart treated by a doctor may be cauterised, frozen with dry ice or removed surgically (never try to do this at home). Some warts left alone disappear without any treatment. Any noticeable change in the shape or size of a wart, or the sudden appearance of several warts should be reported to a medical practitioner.

◌ Use Kombucha tea topically using a cotton wool bud.

☺Apply a small piece of Kombucha poultice over the wart and re-apply twice a day.

A A very level-headed woman reported to us how she had done the above and the wart on her finger disappeared after one week, which seems quite remarkable!

WEIGHT (LOSS AND GAIN)
Gains and losses in weight can provide evidence of someone's state of physical and emotional health. Extra weight adds strain to the organs of the body and can reduce life expectancy, whereas sudden weight loss can be evidence of disease. One has to be sensible in recognising the need to lose weight. Is it for health or fashion reasons? A reducing diet should aim for steady, gradual weight loss. Crash diets are not recommended.

▤ Kombucha can play a significant role in weight reduction, whether as a natural occurrence or as a conscious attempt to lose weight.

▤ In a study in Nigeria researchers fed mice Kargasok Tea (Kombucha) as part of their diet and noted a reduction in food intake and irreversible weight loss. (Hobbs)

▤ Hans Irion (1943) stated - "Through the promotion of the metabolism, unwanted fats and deposits are removed from the body".

∪ As part of a weight reduction diet, allow the Kombucha tea to ferment a little longer until it has become rather sour - but definitely not vinegary. Take a wine-glassful about an hour before meals.

∪ Substitute 1 glass of Kombucha tea for your normal lunch. Kombucha is a nutritious **food** drink containing approximately only 10 calories per fl.oz. when made correctly.

A A correspondent reported, "I have lost 6.4kilos/14lbs in weight while drinking Kombucha without even trying, and my appetite has also diminished".

▤ We have also heard about people with life-threatening diseases, notably cancer and Aids, who have gained weight, some quite substantially, after drinking Kombucha tea.

WHITLOWS (*PARONYCHIA*)
An inflammation of the skin and tissues at the base of the toe or fingernail. Usually caused by a bacterial infection, a whitlow may also be a complication of psoriasis and fungal infections. If not treated it may develop into an abscess.

▤ Kombucha's antiseptic and skin-healing qualities make it an ideal remedy.

☺Apply a small Kombucha poultice to the base of the nail with tape, and replenish daily.

✓Observe cuticle care by periodically pushing it back gently.

CHAPTER 8

FIRST AID WITH KOMBUCHA

NB: These recommendations are no substitute for medical supervision. For serious conditions always consult your health practitioner.

The health advantages of Kombucha have been described in previous chapters in great detail and by now the reader will be quite familiar with its effectiveness used in many different forms. Not only can Kombucha tea be drunk to work at its best from *the inside out*, helping to correct imbalances in the body to make it whole again, but it can also be used very well from *the outside in*, to help conditions where first aid treatment is required.

Every home should possess a good first aid box of course, but often an excellent remedy can be found in the kitchen as well in some natural food form to help a sudden mishap. We are constantly finding new ways of using Kombucha, so when, quite naturally we bump, bruise, burn, blister or get bitten in the course of living, we immediately reach for the Kombucha bottle or jar to help us out. And it does, often, and remarkably well.

For full explanations of Kombucha Recommendations and Symbols, *see* Chapter 7 "A-Z", page 70.

☋ Kombucha Tea - as a drink

◖ Kombucha Tea- applied topically

☺ Kombucha Cream

☺ Kombucha Poultice

◖ Kombucha Compress

◖ Kombucha Bath (full)

◖ Kombucha Foot Bath

◖ Kombucha Steam Inhalation

◖ Kombucha Nasal Spray

To make **Kombucha Vinegar** - *See* Chapter 13, "Kombucha Recipes", p.150.

ABRASIONS

☺Clean the area well with warm water to remove any dirt, and then apply Kombucha tea for bacterial cleansing and healing or apply Kombucha cream. Cover the affected area and secure with a dressing.

ACHING MUSCLES AND JOINTS

☺There is nothing like a Kombucha bath to relieve fatigue. Add 1-2 pints of Kombucha tea or 2 cups of Kombucha vinegar to the water just before entering. Try a self massage over the whole body while you are in the bath, working up from the soles of the feet and squeezing gently and firmly each part of the body, ending with light strokes and smaller circles on the face and head.

ACNE (*See* "A-Z", page 70)

BILIOUS ATTACK

☺Massage Kombucha cream into the area
☋ of the gall bladder under the right lower rib cage, or apply a warm Kombucha compress. Drink Kombucha tea as a daily routine for detoxification and to correct imbalances in the body.

BITES

◖ For superficial bites of domestic or wild animals which harbour germs, wash the wound thoroughly with Kombucha tea and cover with a sterile unmedicated dressing. (NB: Consult your doctor if the bite is more serious or a snake bite).

BLACK EYES

Use a cold dilute Kombucha compress (1:1 with water) to the closed eye and surrounding area and rest. Re-apply as soon as it warms up. Do this for up 15-20 minutes at a time during the course of healing.

BLISTERS

Apply Kombucha tea carefully, using a pad of cotton wool, to bring immediate relief, followed by a Kombucha compress or poultice.

BOILS (*See* "A-Z" - ABSCESS, page 71)

BRUISES

Apply hot and cold Kombucha compresses alternately, using separate cloths, to the bruised and surrounding area.

BUMPS (treat as for BRUISES)

BURNS

For minor burns only - Apply Kombucha tea or Kombucha vinegar topically using a pad of cotton-wool, or use a compress and leave in place. Acts as an antibacterial, will remove smarting, and helps to heal the skin.

CARBUNCLE (treat as for a BOIL)

CATARRH

For immediate relief of congestion, a steam inhalation with Kombucha is effective and will help combat infection. Follow this by massaging the face, paying attention over the nose, sinuses and cheeks using small circular movements which will help drain away excess mucous. Finish with sweeping movements down the face towards the neck.

CHAPPED LIPS

Apply Kombucha tea as often as required to sore and chapped lips, using a pad of cotton-wool or the fingers, or use Kombucha cream.

CHAPPED SKIN (*SEE* CHAPPED LIPS)

CHILBLAINS

If the skin is unbroken, massage with Kombucha cream, using brisk movements to bring localised circulation to the painful area.

Keep extremities warm. (*See* Chap.7, "A-Z" - BLOOD CIRCULATION, page 19)

COLDS

Warmed Kombucha tea is very beneficial to aid respiration, especially when you feel a cold coming on. Try it with ginger - cordial, root or concentrate.

In addition have a Kombucha steam inhalation and Kombucha bath. The inhalation helps to clear congested nasal passages, soothe inflammation and combats infection. The Kombucha bath will aid the process of recovery and help to give you a good night's rest.

COLD SORE (*See* "A-Z" - *HERPES SIMPLEX*, page 87)

CONJUNCTIVITIS

Apply a dilute Kombucha compress (1:1 with water) to the eyelids for 10-15 minutes, keeping eyes closed.

Re-apply 2-3 times per day, as well as drinking Kombucha tea.

CONSTIPATION (*See* "A-Z", page 80)

CORNS

Soak feet in a warm Kombucha foot bath for 20-30 minutes and rub areas firmly with a coarse towel and then a pumice stone. Apply a compress or poultice using Kombucha vinegar at bedtime and first thing in the morning to help soften and the dissolve the corn.

COUGHS

A Kombucha steam inhalation will be good if the cough involves excess mucous or if it is due to a bacterial infection.

A warm Kombucha drink with honey added is also soothing.

CRACKED SKIN

◯ Soak feet in a Kombucha footbath and …

☺Rub Kombucha cream into cracked skin on the heels or hands.

CRAMP (*See "A-Z"*, page 81)

CUTS AND WOUNDS

◯ Apply Kombucha tea immediately to clean the cut or wound and apply a Kombucha compress. Apply a dressing. Renew at least twice daily.

DIARRHOEA (*See "A-Z"*, page 84)

EAR INFECTIONS

◯ The ear is very sensitive and delicate, and an infection can spread rapidly. At the first sign of ear-ache insert a cotton-wool plug which has been dipped in Kombucha tea and apply a warm/hot Kombucha compress to the cheek and ear area. A Kombucha steam inhalation will help combat any infection spreading to the nose and throat. Medical attention should be sought if there is no improvement within 24 hours.

FATIGUE

U A glass of Kombucha tea always seems to give you more energy, especially after a days work. Enjoy a relaxing Kombucha bath or try a foot bath where the beneficial qualities of Kombucha are absorbed quickly via the reflex points to the whole body. Kombucha footbaths are also very beneficial for the elderly or immobile person or on a walking and camping holiday.

GINGIVITIS

◯ Scrupulous attention to mouth hygiene is important in prevention and treatment, using Kombucha tea as a mouth wash, especially after meals and teeth cleaning. Gentle massage of the gums will also speed up healing, using very clean fingers dipped into Kombucha tea and rubbed around the base of the tooth.

This is particularly useful if the gums are too sore to be able to brush.

HANGOVER

U Drink Kombucha tea before a party to prevent a hangover or for a sobering up process afterwards!

HAY FEVER

U Drinking Kombucha tea will help in combating the main problem which is the allergy.

◯ Kombucha steam inhalations are very useful at the first onset of symptoms, such as sneezing, runny nose and streaming eyes. A cool Kombucha compress over the eyes can be soothing and apply Kombucha tea or cream around a sore nose with a cotton-wool pad.

HEADACHE (for MIGRAINE, *see "A-Z"*, page 91)

◯ The source of most headaches is easily traced and a drink of Kombucha tea can
U prove effective in easing one. A cold Kombucha compress can also be applied to the temples and forehead, and a warm compress to the back of the neck. For rapid relief add 4 tablespoons of Kombucha vinegar to 1 pint of boiling water; cover head with a towel and inhale deep breaths. If the cause is catarrhal or sinuses, the steam inhalation will also help combat the infection. Chronic headaches are a strong message of a long-standing complaint of the liver, gall bladder, kidneys or stomach usually, so regular drinking of Kombucha tea would be beneficial.

HEARTBURN

U Sip a cup of warm Kombucha tea slowly with a teaspoon of honey dissolved in it.

☺Rubbing the upper abdomen with Kombucha cream can also help ease discomfort.

HIVES (*See "A-Z"*, page 88)

INDIGESTION (*See also* "A-Z", DIGESTION, page 84)

Drink Kombucha tea to aid digestion before (smaller) meals. If there is extreme discomfort, apply a hot Kombucha compress over the stomach and renew as needed.

INFLUENZA

Take a warm Kombucha bath at the onset, and drink plenty of Kombucha tea to which you could add ginger, lemon and honey. The sick room should be treated with a Kombucha spray to prevent infection spreading.

INSECT BITES

Apply Kombucha tea or vinegar directly to the bite using clean fingers or cotton-wool, re-apply if necessary.

INSOMNIA (*See* "A-Z", page 89)

ITCHING (*See* "A-Z", page 89)

INFLAMMATION

Where there are painful swellings, a hot Kombucha compress will be helpful. With surface inflammation eg. contact dermatitis, bathe with cool Kombucha tea. (For internal inflammation, eg., *See* "A-Z", ARTHRITIS, page 75)

JET-LAG

Drink Kombucha tea before the journey and carry a bottle with you on the flight to help with tiredness, dehydration, cramp and headache.

You can also prepare a Kombucha compress in advance by placing it in a plastic bag and apply to swollen ankles and feet either on the plane or at your journey's end. A Kombucha bath will also help to relax and re-energise you.

LARYNGITIS

Kombucha steam inhalations will ease the breathing, soothe inflammation and help tackle any infection (if this is the cause).

Also drink warm Kombucha tea and add a teaspoonful of honey and a few drops of lemon juice to it.

LUMBAGO

Apply a hot Kombucha compress to the lower back and replace when cold. Repeat three times daily.

Massage lower back and sacrum with Kombucha cream. Rest in bed.

NAPPY RASH

Apply Kombucha cream or Kombucha tea (can be diluted with water 1:1) with a pad of cotton-wool, squeezing out excess moisture. Allow to dry naturally, at every nappy change. Kombucha's pH is similar to the skin and contains natural anti-bacterial agents which will prevent and ease soreness.

NETTLE RASH (URTICARIA)

The simplest method of treatment is to have a lukewarm Kombucha bath, especially if the rash covers a large area of the body. If the area is smaller apply a Kombucha compress or cream. Repeat every few hours until the rash or irritation has cleared. Kombucha tea will help deal with the cause usually connected to allergies, poor immune functioning and stress.

NETTLE STINGS

Is very effectively treated using neat Kombucha tea applied directly to the sting with a pad of cotton-wool or the fingers. This will bring instant coolness and soothing relief, and will prevent the usual hot itching sensation afterwards. Re-apply a second time if necessary.

NEURALGIA

Apply a hot Kombucha compress over the affected area, often the face, which helps reduce inflammation. Replace as it cools down.

Gentle massaging afterwards with Kombucha cream can also help.

NIGHT SWEATS

Apply Kombucha tea topically as a cupped hand bath at bed-time which will greatly assist in preventing night-sweats.

PALPITATIONS

Before going to bed enjoy the relaxation of a Kombucha bath.

RASH (*See* "A-Z", page 95)

RINGWORM

Apply Kombucha tea or vinegar, which is anti-bacterial, at least six times a day, on rising through to bedtime. This will have a healing action and reduce inflammation.

Kombucha cream will also help restore dry flaky patches of skin to normal.

SCIATICA

A cold Kombucha compress can be applied over the area of pain and a warm Kombucha bath will also prove beneficial. The cause needs to be found and corrected, which usually means osteopathic treatment and/or postural correction.

SINUSITIS (*See* "A-Z", page 96)

SORES

Apply a Kombucha compress or poultice to the affected area securing with a dressing.

Kombucha cream can be applied in the later stages of healing.

SORE HANDS

Rinse hands in Kombucha tea, patting off excess moisture and allow to dry naturally, or apply Kombucha vinegar or tea to affected areas with a pad of cotton-wool. Do this daily after a day's work if it is out of doors and hard on the hands, or if they have been in and out of water constantly.

Kombucha cream used any time throughout the day is very beneficial.

SORE THROAT

Gargle frequently with Kombucha tea, or hold it in the mouth for several minutes, and then spitting it out. Kombucha steam inhalations will also ease sore discomfort and deal with any infection.

SPASM

Apply hot Kombucha compresses over the affected area.

Afterwards, while the area is still warm, massage Kombucha cream gently at first and then gradually, as deeply as possible to bring improved circulation to the area.

SPLINTER

Remove the splinter with a sterilised needle or tweezers and apply Kombucha tea or vinegar.

SPRAINS

Use a cold compress immediately (a bag of frozen peas is ideal), to reduce swelling, then apply either a Kombucha compress or poultice to the affected area, replenishing as it dries out. Support the sprain, using a crepe bandage or sling.

SUNBURN

Pat Kombucha tea or vinegar lightly onto the skin with a pad of cotton wool to remove discomfort and promote healing. For larger areas add 1-2 cups of Kombucha vinegar or 1-2 pints of Kombucha tea to a cool/warm bath and soak; then apply Kombucha tea afterwards to areas of need.

Kombucha cream can be used in the later stages to promote healing where the skin is dry and flaking. For serious burns consult your medical practitioner immediately.

THRUSH *(See "A-Z", page 97)*

TOOTHACHE

◊ Rinse the mouth with Kombucha tea holding the liquid in your mouth for up to 5 minutes and then spitting it out. Repeat as often as needed until you can visit your orthodontist. A warm Kombucha compress placed against the skin and over the area of discomfort will also help ease the pain.

TONSILLITIS *(See "A-Z", page 98)*

ULCERS - (MOUTH)

◊ Rinse the mouth frequently with Kombucha tea; also hold a Kombucha-soaked pad in the mouth, against the ulcer in between rinses.

VIRAL INFECTIONS

◊ Kombucha steam inhalations are best given where the respiratory tract and fever are involved

◊ in association with drinking Kombucha tea.

VOMITING

☺ Gently massage Kombucha cream over the stomach

◊ or apply a warm Kombucha compress.

WHITLOWS

☺ Apply a small Kombucha poultice to the base of the nail and apply a dressing. Replenish day and night.

CHAPTER 9

KOMBUCHA FOR PREVENTION OF ILLNESS AND ITS USES WITH CANCER

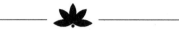

In Britain and in most developed Western countries one in three of the population has or will develop cancer. The numbers are rising: over 300,000 cases a year in the U.K. In the USA, now 40% of the population will contract, but not necessarily die of, cancer. All the significant indicators - incidence, severity and death rate - show it is out of control.

Cancer is a Symptom of the State of our Society:

Some of the causes of cancer are obvious; inhaling nicotine or other noxious fumes, and living too near a major source of electro-magnetic stress (e.g. power transmission lines or microwave towers) or exposure to nuclear radiation. Others are more controversial. The UK government has published findings[1] which show that eating too much red meat causes cancer; but they don't make a distinction between industrially-produced meat which often contains antibiotics, steroids and other nasties, and organic meat which doesn't. Then there's the whole issue of chemicals in all our other foods, many of which will have carcinogenic effects over a long period. Perhaps the most controversial issue is the treatment of our water, which we mentioned in Chapter 6, page 56.

CELL MULTIPLICATION

Body cells divide in order to renew themselves. Sometimes the normal process of cell division gets disrupted and rogue or cancerous cells develop. These are normally quickly recognised and disposed of by a healthy immune system. Rogue cells often multiply as lumps or tumours that are benign (not malignant), but any lump should be examined as soon as possible by a doctor.

Once a malignant tumour has become established, the immune system will attempt to control its growth and will often reverse it. The outcome will depend on whether the weakened immune system that allowed it to become established in the first place can be strengthened. However, if a tumour is not contained, some will eventually spread by a process called metastases to form secondary cancers which are harder to control. The best way to prevent cancer is to have a healthy immune system, and to maintain it.

VARIETIES OF CANCER

Cancer generates a lot of fear because it seems unpredictable - like a lottery. In fact, some cancers can be prevented through a balanced and healthy lifestyle and many, once diagnosed, can be treated. Some cancers are very slow to develop, like prostate cancer. This is common among older men, but they in fact mostly die from another cause. Others have a high rate of recovery - for instance, Hodgkin's Disease (80+%).

Lung cancer comprises almost one third of all cancers. If you don't smoke or live around someone who does, or are not exposed to other forms of airborne pollutants, your chances of getting lung cancer are much less. Breast cancer is a common form of cancer in women. Well established research shows that oestrogen plays a role in breast cancer. Oestrogen is found naturally in the body as a sexual hormone, but also in some plants. However, organic compounds can mimic natural oestrogens, and certain pesticides and plastics are now thought likely to contribute to the higher levels of breast cancer. Cervical and ovarian cancers are also on the increase, but treatable if they are diagnosed early, and there are campaigns to make women more aware of the need for self-examination and of having regular cervical smears.

ENVIRONMENTAL POLLUTION AS A CAUSE OF CANCER
In official quarters, more emphasis is placed on early detection of cancer, than on seeking its causes. In particular, very few studies have been done into the various sources of environmental pollution. The vast majority of industrial chemicals have never been tested for their ability to cause cancer. We know with certainty that animal based foods expose us to organo- and chemo-phosphate pesticides and dioxins which can cause cancer.[2] The safety of drinking water in most parts of the world is open to question, yet this problem is probably seen as an unwelcome time-bomb for any government or official body, and is even avoided by the media. It's high time that we took a much closer personal interest in what chemicals we are exposed to.

VIRUSES OR PARASITES AS CAUSES OF CANCER
Much valuable research has been done by individual doctors all over the world to find a cause for cancer. Many of these see tumours as metabolic disturbances caused by viruses or parasitic fungi. Enderlein[3] and von Brehmer[4] in particular have isolated pathogenic micro-organisms in the blood of cancer patients. Dr. Rudolf Sklenar believed that viruses were involved, and showed how pre-cancerous conditions could be identified by diagnosis of the iris of the patient's eye.[5]

THE CONVENTIONAL TREATMENT OF CANCER
Many people feel that the conventional treatments of cancer, by surgery, chemotherapy and radiotherapy are very harsh on the body. There is, however, no doubt that these treatments save lives. If a tumour is fast growing or quite advanced, it is quite likely that to do nothing about it would soon be fatal. The arguments for chemotherapy or radiotherapy in such cases are quite persuasive. We have close friends whose preference has always been for the 'alternative' route, but whose tumours were so fast growing or advanced that they decided to accept conventional therapy. They insist they would not be alive today if they hadn't received radiotherapy and chemo treatments in conjunction with complementary therapies.

However, if some tumours were diagnosed earlier, it might be possible to avoid the bombardment of harsher treatments. Surely the best course is to nurture our immune system, recognise what fulfils us and makes us happy, and to follow a healthy lifestyle; then our bodies will be more able to provide the natural resistance to the carcinogenic processes which cause cancer.

The Alternative Treatment of Cancer

Some call the alternative approaches to cancer 'the new therapy'. Actually, it is a therapy that comes directly from the 'old model' of Hippocrates - working with Nature! It believes that the body's own immune system is always the best line of defence against disease. Given time and rest, the body usually takes care of disease by itself. If the immune system is for some reason suppressed or our digestive systems are weak, then the sensible course of action must be to find the cause and to help them to become stronger. There is no doubt, as far as alternative approaches to cancer are concerned, that early diagnosis is of paramount importance.

TWO ALTERNATIVE APPROACHES

There are two separate, but connected, approaches to the alternative treatment of cancer. One, the vitamin and diet approach, regards cancer as a nutritional deficiency condition. The other sees it as a chronic, long-standing, metabolic disorder. Much valuable research has been done by individual doctors such as Stanley Gallow (USA), Montagnier (France), and, in Germany, von Brehmer, Schelles, Korner[6], Enderlein and Sklenar.[7] They all see tumours as metabolic disturbances caused by viruses. Enderlein and von Brehmer in particular isolated pathogenic micro-organisms in the blood of their cancer patients.

The effectiveness of Kombucha therapy in containing metabolic disorders has been well established by the German research (*See* "Bibliography", page 173). In addition we discussed in Chapter 3 how Kombucha stabilises the blood chemistry and the intestinal flora, both of which actions will have an immediate effect on immune health. Lastly, the presence of lactic acid in Kombucha tea in its most beneficial form, as L+lactic acid, is significant. It is never found in the tissues of people with cancer, and its lack has been established as indicating susceptibility to cancer.

THE MOST EFFECTIVE WAY IS PREVENTION

Kombucha therapy's effectiveness as a prophylactic was confirmed in the early 1950s by the research of the Soviet government which found that Kombucha-drinking communities were protected from the cancer epidemic caused by wartime over-production of toxic materials in the trans-Ural industrial heartland.

Kombucha used on its own is an excellent preventative of cancer because:
• it helps to establish a balanced and healthy intestinal flora
• it keeps the body from building up toxins and other waste products
• it encourages balanced metabolic function
• its acidity will discourage pathogenic micro-organisms in the blood

PIONEERS OF CANCER TREATMENT WITH KOMBUCHA

Dr.Rudolf Sklenar felt that every chronic disease is triggered by a metabolic malfunction which results in an accumulation of waste products in the body and an environment in which a virus can develop. He used to say, "no cancer patient has a healthy digestive tract!" It was this belief that prompted him to experiment with Kombucha therapy on his cancer patients, and he had surprisingly good results.[8] These may, in part, have been due to his ability to diagnose cancer early, when Kombucha has the best opportunity to build up the immune function.

Dr.Sklenar wrote in 1986:

"During the more than 30 years I have been working as a general practitioner I have been using, for therapy, the beverage prepared from the tea fungus Kombucha, and also the drops of the Kombucha concentrate, preferably combining it with coli preparations to cure intestinal disturbances.

"The therapeutics based on Kombucha produced good therapeutic results in cases of metabolic diseases, also with those of a chronic nature. Good results were achieved also with cancer diseases in various stages. In no instance undesired side effects or late effects caused by a treatment with these therapies was ascertainable."

Dr Veronika Carstens, a distinguished doctor (and daughter of a former German president), also used Kombucha therapy with cancer patients in her medical practice.

A specialist who runs Kombucha House in Australia, Veronica Perko, advises that cancer patients could well drink up to a full litre of Kombucha tea, spread over 24 hours. The first glassful should be drunk on rising, well before breakfast, and others can be after meals.

ARE THERE CERTAIN KINDS OF PEOPLE AT HIGHER RISK OF CANCER?

As we see in Chapter 11, there are many factors which contribute towards total health besides our physical condition. Profiles of cancer patients have been studied to see if certain personality types are more likely to get cancer. At the Bristol Cancer Help Centre we found that a large percentage of cancer patients were very creative people who had not been able to develop their creativity to the full. We also found that many were very kind and giving individuals who put their own needs last, while others were suppressed and were not in touch with their real feelings, especially their anger and resentment.[9]

Clearly a high level of stress can create an environment in the body in which cancer cells may take hold, because traumas depress the immune system. The death of a loved one, a business failure or deep personal loss or shock, can trigger malignancy to start, though it may not surface for several years. This is why it is important to come to terms with these traumas at an emotional level within a reasonable time, through counselling, a good listening doctor or complementary therapist or sharing with close friends. Holding these wounds inside is not good for the body!

Pawpaw and Essiac as Cancer Treaments

Through our work with Kombucha we have been introduced to two quite remarkable herbal treatments for cancer from two different ancient cultures. These two products taken in combination with Kombucha have given significant results for people with cancer who have reported improved energy, quality of life and reversal of tumour growth, even in some serious cancer conditions. Kombucha , pawpaw and Essiac can be taken in conjunction with orthodox cancer treatments, but please check with your doctor first.

PAW PAW

Pawpaw's genuine health benefits have been brought to the world's attention by the aborigines of Australia, whose medicines are connected to the earth's true riches. Pawpaw is a delicious tropical fruit well known for its nutritional qualities and as an aid to the digestion of proteins. Tests now conducted in Australia have found that it has additional value in alleviating cancer.[10]

In 1962, Stan Sheldon was dying from lung cancer when he heard about an aborigine remedy using pawpaw leaves. He made a daily supply of tea from fresh leaves and stems - filling a pan with leaves, covering them with water, and simmering for two hours before straining the liquid. He drank about 20-mls three times a day.

After two months, he went for a compulsory chest x-ray as part of the then current tuberculosis control programme. Both lungs were entirely clear of disease - cancer as well as TB. He told his doctors that he no longer had cancer, and they didn't believe him - until they did their own tests. Then they recommended that he continue drinking the pawpaw leaf tea. Mr Sheldon who is now over 90 years old, has passed on the recipe to other cancer victims.

Pawpaw works well with Kombucha, and preparations made in Australia are available. Normally the fruit, seed, stem and leaves are used in the concentrated extract. You can also get the extract combined with Kombucha, but there would be no need if you make your own Kombucha beverage. (*See* "Resources Section and Suppliers")

ESSIAC - THE RENE CAISSE HERBAL MIXTURE

The other herbal remedy is one that has been used by the Ojibway Indians of Canada for centuries as a treatment for cancer. A nurse, Rene Caisse, was given the recipe by an elderly patient who had recovered years earlier from breast cancer using only this remedy. For nearly 60 years she treated thousands of cancer patients successfully, refusing to accept any payment. She became a cause celebre in 1940 when the Canadian Government effectively closed her down, in spite of a petition being raised to prevent it containing 55,000 signatures, from doctors, friends and many former patients. Rene Caisse died at the age of 70 after dedicating half a century to what she called "suffering humanity", and still without recognition of her remedy.

Essiac (an anagram of Caisse) is a mixture of four herbs: burdock root, sheep sorrel, slippery elm and Turkish rhubarb root. These herbs are known to be effective in attacking and breaking down tumours, oxygenating and purifying the blood, eliminating toxic waste, strengthening the organs and mucous membranes and stimulating the growth of new cells. They also contain large quantities of essential vitamins and minerals. The herbal formula has been kept alive by word of mouth and now thankfully can be obtained quite easily. Some suppliers over-charge, but we give sources which provide it at a reasonable price. Essiac can also be used in conjunction with Kombucha. In fact, many people have found that, with advanced cases of cancer, Essiac, pawpaw and Kombucha may all be used beneficially together. One way to test which, and how much to use, is by muscle testing (*See* page 51).

REFERENCES

1   *The Daily Telegraph*, 5th Sept, 1997

2   Steingraber, Sandra, *Living Downstream: An Ecologist looks at Cancer and the Environment*: Addison Wesley (Merloyd Lawrence), 1997.

3   Enderlein, Prof. Dr. Gunter, *Akmon*, vol.1, nos.1- 1955, 2- 1957 & 3- 1959, Ibica, Aumuhle/Hamburg.

4   von Brehmer, Dr. Wilhelm, *Siphonospora polymorpha*: Link, Haag.

5   Sklenar, Dr. Rudolf, *Krebsdiagnose aus dem Blut und die Behandlung von Krebs un Prakanzerosen mit der Kombucha und Colipraparaten* (Cancer diagnosis through the blood and the treatment of cancer and pre-cancerous ailments by means of Kombucha and colicines): Fasching, Klangenfurt, 1983.

6   Korner, H., "Ein Parasit im Blut" (A parasite in the blood): *Raum & Zeit*, no.19, 1985.

7   Sklenar, *op.cit.*

8   Sklenar, *op.cit.*

9   Thompson, Dr. Rosy, *Loving Medicine: Patients' Experiences of the Bristol Cancer Help Centre*: Gateway 1989.

10 Tietze, Harald, *Paw Paw as Healing Medicine*: Phree Books, Australia.

CHAPTER 10

IN-DEPTH CASE HISTORIES

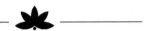

There is an abundance of research available on Kombucha, mostly from German and Russian sources, including chemical analyses and accounts of its use in clinical trials in connection with various illnesses.

What has been lacking is a body of case histories that can make up a more human picture of how Kombucha has helped with a wide variety of illnesses. As it is a nutritious food and an energy medicine, it is more appropriately studied from a holistic viewpoint, taking into account the patient's whole life situation and history, rather than from the more limited symptomatic approach of allopathic medicine. Symptoms which are suppressed by medication may lie dormant, building up and adding to the picture of disease and imbalance within the body.

We are including these case histories to encourage people to persevere with Kombucha, as so often we give up if an instant healing is not achieved. Many illnesses take years or a lifetime to develop, therefore some patience is needed for changes and lasting improvements to take place with Kombucha therapy, though many people do experience beneficial effects straight away. The people who generously agreed to be interviewed as case studies for this book are all part of the Kombucha Network and have willingly supplied information about their progress. We have tried to take into account other remedies and medications that they were taking, to give a more balanced picture.

These are human stories of people whose courage, intelligence and patience have been rewarded with significant improvement in their health. They are living examples of how we can start to take responsibility for our own health, and we hope that they will inspire you to pursue the path of self-empowerment. Regretably, when some of the people in these case histories told their doctors that they were taking Kombucha and experiencing improvements they received little encouragement. Some doctors were hostile while others were only tacitly supportive. Our hope is that, in the future, it might be possible to include positive feedback from some patients' doctors too.

Multiple Sclerosis is a debilitating disease that has uneven distribution, with one of the highest incidences being in Britain. It causes great suffering to individuals and their families because it affects mostly people in their 20s and 30s. The attacks usually become progressive, leading to increased loss of muscular function through the build-up of plaques in the myelin sheaths of the central nervous system. To date orthodox medicine has found no cure for M.S..

BOB BANHAM

(aged 44) was first diagnosed as having M.S. in 1986, although he had a number of symptoms the year before. This is how he describes his involvement with Kombucha tea:

"At first I just experienced odd pains and numbness in various parts of the body, but this soon degenerated into the classic symptoms of M.S.: blurred/double vision, urgency and/or inability to urinate, sudden loss of balance and strength in the legs, and then ultimately the inability to walk at all without my wife's support.

"I had been involved in martial arts for the previous twenty years and in 1982 had commenced a three year clinical training in acupuncture and Western herbalism. As well as studying Chinese herbal medicine and homoeopathy, I had also learned Transcendental Meditation, and in 1985 spent several months in the Far East, specifically the Philippines and Australia, studying acupuncture, native herbalism and other traditional healing systems. Since I was about 17 years old I have been smoking cannabis on a fairly regular basis.

"All this I see as a grounding for what I was going to have to do over the next ten years. I actually think I was being 'set up'. Upon diagnosis, I was offered ACTH injections by my GP which I declined. I have in the past eleven year since my diagnosis received no treatment of any kind from conventional Western medicine, but as you will see from the above, I had a very clear direction in which to look for help.

"I spent the next 7-8 years searching for anything within the fields of natural medicine which might be of value. I looked at acupuncture, of course. I had experience with M.S. in this field as I had in the past treated three or four sufferers. I looked at herbal medicine, both Western and Chinese. I looked at Ayurveda (traditional Indian medicine), aromatherapy, reflexology, kinesiology, diet, health supplements, exercise, yoga and yogic-type breathing exercises and, of course, meditation and visualisation.

"I managed to devise a programme which enabled me to start walking properly again, allowed me to continue teaching martial arts and to practise acupuncture, albeit at a more leisurely pace - and then I discovered Kombucha.

"I first started drinking Kombucha in 1993-4, after being given a culture by a friend who knew very little about it. He didn't know that it was said to benefit M.S., and I had no more than a bad photocopy of some hand-written instructions for brewing.

"We then discovered that there was anecdotal evidence that Kombucha could help in cases of M.S., but there was no information on dosage, so I started drinking about a pint a day to see what would happen. Quite quickly there was a very pronounced detoxifying effect - headache, bad breath, feeling 'spaced-out', etc - which I recognise from fasting, and then things began to settle down.

"It was after drinking Kombucha daily for four months that my wife said 'I think you seem to have a little more energy; I wonder if it's the Kombucha?' To be honest, I hadn't noticed any difference or, if I had, I wasn't placing too much importance on it, in case it was just imagination or wishful thinking. It's very easy to clutch at any straw that drifts within reach, and I had always resisted that impulse.

"Anyway, I knew that the only way to be sure was to see what happened when I stopped, and then to start drinking it again and note any changes. Well, there were definite differences within a week of stopping my daily dose of the 'magic brew'. Energy levels dropped, physical ability declined and psychologically I felt a lot less positive, almost apathetic. After two weeks I started back on it and, within a week or so this time, I started to notice improvements again.

"I have spoken at some length to the Myelin Trust (one of the support organisations for M.S.), and they recommend a starting dose of 1 teaspoonful three times a day, because some people with M.S. are very weak and sensitive. I have never taken less than three good-sized glasses a day (about 1-1½ pints; 300 -450-mls), and have never experienced any adverse effects after that first time." [detoxification is very individual; we suggest that the recommended dose be followed, after first building up from smaller amounts. Ed.]

"Since joining the Kombucha Network, we have provided cultures to people with M.S. in Britain and all over Europe, and I see my next job as collating the experiences of these people and putting together the result in a form which will allow the medical profession to take this ancient gift seriously. It has helped to change my life, or at least has helped me to deal with the changes life has thrust upon me, and I know that I am not alone.

"I stop taking Kombucha periodically for a week or so every couple of months now, as I think it is important as with any medicine, to allow the body to normalise and to let one assess the effects. I want to stress that I have no concerns whatever about its use in M.S. management, or with any other health problem; or if it is used just as a tonic, a detoxifier or an energy booster. I think most adverse criticism comes from people or organisations who would like to make money from it, but realise they can't in the U.K.. Tough!

"One other use I have found for Kombucha is horticultural. We know that the reason it is so valuable in the treatment of candidiasis is because it is acidic, and most moulds, mildews, fungi, etc, don't like that. I had an extremely bad case of white mildew on the leaves of my courgettes and ridge cucumbers. It was so bad I was about to throw them away. I sprayed the leaves with Kombucha liquid and the next morning they were clear. A week later they were strong, healthy and producing fruit like crazy!"

Bob is one of our dedicated regional coordinators on the Kombucha Tea Network UK. We send him all the enquiries from M.S. sufferers which he personally answers. He encloses a personalised letter of encouragement with cultures that he sends out to enquirers on the Network with M.S. To date he has supplied about 500 people. Bob is conducting a survey of these people, with the support of the coordinator of the Neurological Support Services of the National Health Service, and will publish the results in due course.

Women are often more open about health matters than men. In this case, it was the mother, with reasonably good health, who persuaded her family to try drinking Kombucha for their health problems.

DIANE THOMAS

(aged 55), started brewing and drinking Kombucha herself in 1995, and felt well on it. "No doubt due to my advancing years and the menopause, I had been experiencing stiff joints, especially when I got out of bed in the morning. Drinking Kombucha tea regularly seems to have eased the stiffness, and this is now no longer a problem."

Roger, her husband (aged 56), has been an insulin-dependent **diabetic** for 30 years and was horrified at the idea of taking something with so much sugar used in the making, but was persuaded that the sugars are converted into organic acids. He started gingerly with only one glass of Kombucha a day, but is now willingly taking up to two glasses more, due to the improvement that he is experiencing. He monitors his sugar levels carefully, and has been able, in just over a year, to reduce his insulin intake from 28 units to 17. He leads a very active life, and feels very well on his reduced dose. The hospital is also very pleased with his progress.

Francesca, Diane's daughter (aged 30), has had very bad **eczema** which started as patches over her body in childhood but, in her mid-20s, became critical; her whole body was covered. Cortisone creams helped a little, but it was hard for her to apply the cream all over. She tried acupuncture without effect, and Chinese herbalism, which helped a little. The eczema was so extreme that some days she couldn't even get out of bed because she was so depressed with the state of her body.

Francesca started drinking two glasses of Kombucha a day in early 1996, and the first thing she noticed was that she could "see more clearly". She has always had good vision, but on first taking Kombucha tea the energy boost made everything seem brighter and clearer. The eczema at first seemed to get worse, but she persisted with Kombucha, and it disappeared gradually over a period of about a year. Francesca temporarily stopped drinking Kombucha during pregnancy and found small patches recurring. However, the fact that her eczema is now under control has done wonders for her self-confidence and, of course, her depression has lifted also.

Anthony, Diane's son (aged 27), has had **asthma** since he was 8 years old. He takes one glass of Kombucha a day (masked by Ribena, because he doesn't like Kombucha's taste). It has helped him to cope better. He uses his inhaler less now, but his mother thinks he could do even better if he had a more positive attitude!   Diane recalls, "My interest in alternative methods began about fifteen years ago when Anthony developed an extremely lethargic condition after having a viral illness. I had had exactly the same thing - it was a flu-type cold. I recovered, but Anthony, who was a healthy thirteen year old boy at the time, rosy-cheeked, bright-eyed, energetic and cheerful, became a grey-skinned, dull eyed, stooped 'old man' who did not have enough energy to climb the stairs. This was before the terms 'M.E.' and 'Post-viral Syndrome', were widely used. Anthony could not go to school; his whole life fell apart and, what was worse, our doctor was unsympathetic, even aggressively dismissive. He suggested seeing a psychiatrist - no doubt he felt powerless.

"Meanwhile Anthony missed 12 months of school and became very depressed. Instinctively I turned to things over which I had some control, such as what he ate. I switched to a wholefood diet with plenty of fruit and fresh vegetables, cutting out all tinned, packed and convenience food. I also gave him plenty of vitamins and minerals. Gradually he improved. After two years from the onset of his illness we began hearing about M.E. (Chronic Fatigue Syndrome). We think that's what he must have had. The experience left me disillusioned with conventional medicine. I wish I had known about Kombucha then."

RICHARD KOTCH

is a yoga teacher (aged 26). In 1996 he went to India to study, but that October, became very ill with a potentially-lethal viral fever. He came home for treatment. After a number of blood tests he was diagnosed as having **M.E. (Chronic Fatigue Syndrome)** He had all the unpleasant symptoms of this condition, i.e. chronic fatigue, headache, dizziness, poor sleeping, flu-like symptoms and depression. In November 1996 he was given a culture by a Kombucha Network coordinator and started drinking the beverage.

He began taking more than the maximum amount of Kombucha tea recommended - i.e. a tumblerful 3 times a day instead of the normal wineglass. Richard noticed an instant improvement in his condition which continued for about five months and then seemed to level off.

We asked him how he knows that it is Kombucha that has helped him?

1. He says he uses the empty bucket theory. This means that when you have no energy - in other words, an empty bucket - then you can easily tell when a new amount of energy has been added, whereas when you have a 3/4 full bucket to start with, it's more difficult to tell.

2. He is taking two other health products - Aloe Vera and Blue Green Algae. However, when he stops taking either of these two for one or two days he doesn't notice any change in the way he feels, but when he stops taking Kombucha he really notices the difference, i.e. his energy declines.

Richard says, "Having M.E. has made me very aware of my body's energy and the remedies and treatments which have been most effective. Kombucha has the most dramatic effect. It is by far the cheapest (compared to Aloe Vera and Blue Green Algae which are both expensive supplements) and has proved to be the most effective."

Richard has coped with moving house recently and currently manages to teach two or three yoga classes per week now.

LYNNE THOMPSON

is a Northumbrian who has always lived in the countryside and she learned to ride her grandfather's Clydesdales before she could walk. Lynne has always been around horses, and for many years used to look after racehorses while also running a pub. Now involved with less demanding 'event' horses, she still rides every day.

Lynne's main health problems have been debilitating **allergies** and, more seriously, **asthma**. Her childhood allergies were so bad that she had a medical desensitising at the age of 19. This helped with the allergies a little, but unfortunately, within four years, she developed asthma which got progressively worse over the next 20 years. Over that period she was dependent on at least one Ventolin inhaler a week and for the past five years also on the steroid drug Pulmicort.

Three years ago, after a serious chest infection, Lynne developed **M.E**, with dramatic weight loss, nodules on her hands, and hair loss. She also has **Sjogren's Syndrome** which resulted in dry mouth and eyes. In June 1996 her boyfriend's father, who is a health enthusiast, gave her some Kombucha tea, and, at the age of 43, her life started changing. Her asthma stopped dramatically, almost at once, and she soon discarded for good both the inhalers and the steroids, to the astonishment of her doctor, who insists she must continue on Kombucha therapy. She had regularly experienced six to seven **chest infections** a year for the past eight years. These have also ceased, to her great relief. Her hair, which had become quite thin, has also much improved.

Since starting Kombucha therapy Lynne now no longer suffers from **hay fever**. In previous years, she has always been affected by the bright yellow flowers of oilseed rape crops.

In spite of the immediate improvement to her asthma, Lynne recognises that there is so much in her body that has been out of balance and that she must be patient. She has great faith in Kombucha, which has become a natural part of her diet. Lynne had always driven herself, and wouldn't listen to her doctor's pleas to slow down. Recently, however, she has given up work, realising that she must give her body a chance to heal properly. Lynne has been drinking $\frac{1}{2}$ -pint of Kombucha tea every day after lunch. She says she will now try drinking a wine glass three times a day, which is the recommended amount and frequency and is more beneficial for the body than just one large glass a day. She also uses Kombucha as a mouth rinse for her Sjögren's dry mouth symptom. She has three batch brewing bowls on the go in her airing cupboard at a time.

Archie, her boyfriend, drinks the same amount once a day at present and has found that his **itchy scalp** and **dandruff** problems are much eased. He rubs the beverage into the itchy spots, and also uses it as a hair rinse. Their 7 year-old Doberman dog had always suffered with **skin problems**, so they gave him bits of the Kombucha culture to eat daily in his food, and his coat is now much better.

Some of the most useful research into uses of Kombucha is being conducted by people in great need who work by instinct.

EVE MYERS,

(aged 56) is a Yorkshire woman living on Tyneside. Eve has endured a lifetime of ill health. She has been plagued with **defective thyroid** function, for over 40 years and has been dependent on thyroxin tablets. Her symptoms include **skin problems**, such as sore cracks cellulitis, and an **auto-immune disease** which brings the added risk of abscesses developing under the skin.

Eve has had a **weight problem** for years, aggravated by general **fluid retention** which has been particularly troublesome in her legs. She has had **asthma** for many years which has created difficulties with her attempts to develop her singing voice. Latterly she has also had **fluid on her lungs**. In the last four years Eve has developed **glaucoma**, a serious and painful eye condition caused by faulty fluid emission behind the eye. She has been treated with eye drops containing cortisone and steroids, two powerful drugs which are not friendly to the body's metabolism.

In November 1996, Eve fell awkwardly onto a bicycle pedal which grazed her lower leg near the ankle. It became ulcerated and infected, resulting in an inch-long angry and pitted wound. This was a vascular, **venous ulcer**, a hard one to heal. Her first course of antibiotics was ineffective. Then she was given penicillin which affected her stomach badly, so Eve gave up on antibiotics. In addition, her wound was dressed with viscopaste bandages (zinc impregnated) which, unfortunately, always seemed to tear off some of the wound when they were removed. The pain was unbearable, and she had little confidence in the nurse who changed her dressings every two days. This all affected her life; she couldn't drive her car without pain, or walk any distance. She tried to change the dressings herself, but just couldn't manage.

Quite beside herself, some four months later, and feeling she could get no help from doctors or hospitals, Eve confided in a friendly assistant pharmacist in her local chemists. The pharmacist mentioned that she brewed Kombucha, gained great personal benefit from drinking it, and said she had read that the culture could be used to good effect as a poultice on the skin. She gave Eve one to try. As directed, Eve put it directly on the wound, and covered it with dressings and a tubular bandage. She found that it smarted quite a lot for 10 minutes, and then it eased a bit. She persevered, and within 90 minutes the pain had been replaced by a warm, comforting glow.

A few hours later, after a second application, the wound had gone down, but the skin around it had started to blister. She realised that maybe she should not have used the Kombucha culture neat. Because of its sponge-like form, the liquid contained in it is concentrated and very acidic. However, when the dressing came off this time, the infection seemed to have drained out of the wound and the swelling had gone. Eve's experimentation became more inventive, and aware that her skin was very fragile, she soaked a culture next time in water for 12 hours and squeezed out the excess liquid before putting it on the wound. She anointed the skin around the wound with Kanillosan, a camomile-based viscous ointment which keeps the skin protected, and after five days of Kombucha application, the purple-coloured skin around the wound lost its puffiness and the infection cleared completely.

During this time, Eve was taking no drugs, except painkillers. The remarkable thing was that, within a week of applying the Kombucha culture externally, the fluid on her lungs also disappeared and has not returned. In addition she lost 10 pounds in weight, and two inches off her hips. Kombucha was proving to be more effective by far than the diuretics she used to take, which had only limited effect on the water retention.

Eve's skin has now become clear and soft, and the wound has closed so completely that it looks as if it will be scar-free. Eve started making Kombucha tea herself three weeks after the ulcer treatment and she will monitor the effects now of taking it internally.

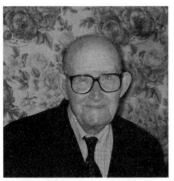

Tom Robinson, Centinarian

TOM ROBINSON

reached his 100th birthday just before this book was published. He was invalided from the First World War after two bouts of rheumatic fever and suffered from this fever again, which he knows can be life-threatening to many, twice during the Second World War. He has outlived two wives, a son and daughter, and has several grandchildren and great grandchildren. Three years ago, he began to experience great difficulty in eating. The **skin** in his throat had become **over-sensitive**, causing him great discomfort and pain when he tried to swallow, and ended up only being able to have liquid foods. Tom is a man who values his independence, brewing beer and growing all his own vegetables. He continued to dig his garden well into his 90s. The discomfort he was experiencing in his throat affected his **sleep**, and as he hadn't slept well for years, he became quite depressed at the bleak outlook ahead. Life didn't seem worth living.

In January 1995 a man who does a grocery van round took Tom a bottle of Kombucha tea to try. Within ten days he found that the pain had gone and he could swallow more easily and was consequently sleeping better. He insisted on getting a fungus to brew for his own needs and also to give away to his friends. Soon he was supplying other people on the sheltered-housing estate where he lives. People were amazed how his **energy** had improved and his **digestion** was better. Tom found that he was soon able to start digging his garden again.

Then, a year later, Tom fell and broke his thighbone; he was hospitalised for a month. He felt that he was not given the physiotherapy he needed to give him confidence to move around at home on his own. He fell again, breaking the same bone, and spent another month in hospital, this time having three screws inserted to stabilise the bone. When Tom got home the second time, he worked hard at building up his leg's strength by walking daily round the block, assisted by a frame with wheels. But Tom found it difficult now to carry his 3-litre brewing bowl in and out of the airing cupboard, and gave up Kombucha brewing, but not before he had stored some six bottles in his fridge.

Alick went to see him in June 1997, a year after his second return from hospital, and found that he was still having the occasional little eggcupful of Kombucha from these bottles, trying to spin out what he had. The healing of his throat had continued well. Tom didn't like being dependent on others cooking for him when he came out of hospital. He felt he also couldn't ask anyone to brew Kombucha for him either. Alick solved the problem by equipping Tom with an electric heating tray for fermenting his Kombucha tea. This has been placed on his kitchen worktop, making it more manageable for him to use than his airing cupboard. Tom is thrilled that he can brew his own Kombucha again.

Tom resists going to the doctor and says that he "doesn't believe in medicines". But he does believe in the healing power of Nature and feels that "we should return to some of the old natural remedies which would help us more than the drugs we depend on now". He remembers how, when he was young and living in Bristol, many people could not afford to go to the doctor. Instead they got their remedies from a local herbalist. Tom, who has good eyesight, hearing and memory, has been a gardener for most of his life and still grows all his own vegetables, though, since his thigh operations, he has to have help with the digging. He says that he lives cheaper than anyone else in his village His other secrets of long life are that he always eats a light meal in the evening, followed by a beer and a whisky.

JAN ROBINSON

worked in a commercial bank in London in a demanding public relations job, which she did not find self-fulfilling. Already interested in yoga, which she taught, Jan went on to train in Shiatsu, starting her practice in 1991. In 1992, after many tests, she was finally diagnosed with **M.E. (Chronic Fatigue Syndrome)**. Jan who had been driving herself too hard, had to stop work completely. She tried 18 months of psychotherapy, but this did not help, and she realised that living in London was just too stressful for her. In 1994 she moved to Bristol to be with her partner.

Jan's partner Tim had heard about Kombucha through the Internet, but could not find how to get hold of a culture until he met Alick on a weekend course. Jan started drinking Kombucha in 1995, and within two weeks noticed an improvement in her energy. She reports:

"The improvement I noticed when I began drinking Kombucha was in my **digestion** - I felt that I was absorbing more from my food. The muscle wasting that I had experienced started to reverse, and I began to feel physically stronger. Drinking Kombucha also had a diuretic effect on me which I managed to balance by not drinking Kombucha late at night, and taking no more than half a glass a day in total. I add a little warm water to it to take the chill off, because I cannot drink or eat anything cold from the fridge as it affects my digestion. I add ginger to the Kombucha brew, which is warming for me, particularly in winter. My **abdominal scar** diminished when I used Kombucha as a poultice. I also got rid of a small cyst on my eye in the same way."

"I do suffer from immune deficiency, but to call it M.E. is an oversimplification as in my case there are many other factors involved - hormonal, digestive, allergic, spiritual, etc. Although my energy level has improved, I cannot count on any set amount of active time each day, because it is still very variable, but I average about four 'active' hours a day. I could not honestly say that Kombucha alone is responsible for my overall improvement, because I am working with many other healing factors, including Chinese and Western herbal medicine, Qi Gong, meditation, acupuncture, Bach Flower remedies, yoga, etc. So I feel it is the combined approach that is successful."

Jan makes her beverage with green tea and either elderflower, hibiscus, jasmine or ginger added to it.

BARBARA BRUCE

(aged 60) says her Kombucha experience has given her a new lease of life.

"I have had a life-long history of **indifferent kidney function** which was revealed through 'camel-like' qualities of **water retention**, and of painful **rheumatism** which I believe came from a build-up of toxins in the muscles. Conventional medicine had given me some relief but, in my late 20s, I had a horrendously painful experience with prescribed medications. I looked to other ways of bringing relief. Exercise, especially swimming, encouraged my kidney function. A diet from which white sugar and white flour were excluded, but which included organic food, and finally a vegetarian diet, all certainly helped. Although naturally slim, my body was often quite distended. It was an effort to maintain some quality of life. An osteopath gave much valued assistance, but advised me to start saving for a **hip replacement**, as my hip was becoming very painful.

"I would go as far as to say that I was 'saved by Kombucha'. In 1994, a friend gave me a culture and explained how to make it. I drank ¼-pint three times a day and within two weeks noticed considerable changes. Kidney function was much improved and the distension around the middle and the belly just subsided. After swimming one day, I noticed that there was no usual increase in kidney function. Quite obviously the kidneys were functioning more normally! To my surprise, I realised there was also no pain in my hip. A recent check by a chiropractor indicated that it was fine, and certainly no hip replacement was indicated.

"Kombucha seems to help where it is needed. An unexpected benefit has been improved vision. When there was a mix-up between old and new glasses, I was surprised to discover I could read with the old glasses, and have not needed the regular changes in prescription that I used to have.

"I have found Kombucha to be an energy booster. Experience has taught me to respect the power of Kombucha. On one occasion, a new batch of the brew tasted so good that I drank three times the usual amount. As a result, my kidneys went into overdrive, and I had a great thirst. It is advisable also not to drink Kombucha continuously, but to take breaks for periods in between. So far I have resisted the temptation to take Kombucha with me on holiday. However, I do find that by the third week my kidney function noticeably slows down, and that my energy lessens. As a result, Kombucha is the first drink I have on my return.

"To quote a book title 'The Healing Power of Illness' - I believe in the paradox that illness heals. It does so by the mind working through the body to show us what we need to learn about ourselves, so that the spirit can progress too, for we are body, mind and spirit. By following Kombucha therapy, we are taking responsibility for ourselves, claiming back our own power and seeking information and experience for ourselves, which is very different from believing that others will heal us.

"I do brew for others. A popular recipe is: a teaspoon of organic green tea and 2 teabags of Dr Stuart's Botanical Teas (such as alpine strawberry) left for five days. Delicious drinks are made by topping up the 150mls/1-wine glass (US: ¾-cup) of Kombucha with either orange or lemon juice. This tastes especially good as the first drink of the day.

"From my own experience, I recommend Kombucha strongly. I also urge that if you listen to your own body and use your intuition, you should get a feeling of what you need. Some people drink Kombucha only for a short time and feel they don't need it any longer. It is good to take responsibility for yourself. Should you feel the need to start again, a new culture can be provided.

"Kombucha is the modern drink from ancient times - so we can adopt the thinking of the New Age, taking responsibility for our own lives."

Dr Rudolph Sklenar was a German doctor who did much research on the benefits of Kombucha therapy for cancer patients. We felt, therefore, that it would be of interest to hear how someone suffering from **cancer** has got on with her Kombucha treatment.

ISABEL SHAW,

(aged 73) is an artist who, up until two years ago, enjoyed a career teaching adults. Her two children are also artists. She has taught drawing and painting in technical colleges and in teacher training colleges. Isabel has also privately taken many commissions from the Royal Horticultural Society for paintings of wild flowers in watercolour, and was awarded several of their medals. Her interest in wild flowers arose from her concern about their destruction due to chemical farming methods. At a recent sale of paintings and sculpture which she helped to organise in her home town of Holmfirth, she and her colleagues raised £23,000 for the Macmillan Nurses who work with cancer patients in the UK. Isabel has sold her own paintings in this Macmillan Cancer Relief Exhibition every year since the first, 30 years ago.

Isabel has been used to having lots of energy, but she has also had her share of stress. Her husband had a stroke, followed by epilepsy, four years before he died. During this period, his behaviour was very unpredictable, and he became quite dependent on her.

Isabel fire-watched in Liverpool which suffered severe bombing in the Second World War - and it was then, she says, that she started smoking. "Doctors used to recommend it then, she says, for soothing the nerves, and nearly everyone I knew smoked! I managed to give it up for five years until my mother died in 1965. Then, I found I couldn't sleep and didn't want to eat either; I just wanted to smoke. I managed to stop smoking again about a year before I was diagnosed with **lung cancer** in 1995."

Isabel had the conventional treatment of chemo- and radiotherapy with its unpleasant side effects. The cancer site disappeared but, as she says, she has the 'small-cell' variety of cancer, which can reappear anywhere. Last year (1996) it reappeared in the lymph glands at the base of her neck. In June 1996 she was in hospital with a **thrombosis** for which she is still taking warferin treatment .

In October she started chemotherapy for this secondary cancer, which affected her appetite badly. In December she was introduced to a Yorkshire healing centre and asked for their help which she greatly values and feels has helped to realign her body's energies. They introduced her to Kombucha, which she has been brewing for herself since then.

The healers advised Isabel to take Essiac also, a specific herbal mixture developed as a cancer treatment by the native Ojibway Indians in Canada, with Paw Paw extract which is well known in Australia as the aborigines' cure for cancer, together with Kombucha. (*See* Pawpaw and Essiac as Cancer Treatments, p.110, and "Resources Section and Supplies") "At this point I decided to go flat out to help myself, believing that it is better to do something for oneself rather than do nothing". Isabel takes them together first thing in the morning, before breakfast, after lunch and after supper.

"I can say that, as far as I know, the cancer does not seem to have spread to other parts of my body as it could well have done by now. I am sure that Kombucha has helped to keep up my energy levels and counter some of the effects of the chemotherapy drugs. I have also been able to eat a wider range of foods than was possible in the last couple of years.

"I know there are no guarantees in this life, and there is no definite proof of how effective Kombucha, Paw Paw and Essiac have been in arresting my condition. However, I do know for certain that I would not want to stop taking them, They produce no side effects and will not damage me, and there is much to be said for that. Without the help and care I have received from conventional medicine, from my splendid healers, and from the natural therapies, I would not be here now."

JOHN & ENID DAVIES

live in North Wales, and John has been a **diabetic** since 1981, and has been taking orthodox medications for this. Enid (aged 65) had **rheumatic fever** when she was 15, and has suffered from **oedma** in her legs ever since, treating this with acupuncture and homoeopathy. John, who is 72, started having **blood clots** in his right leg which led to the big toe of his foot having to be amputated in 1993. In 1995 trouble with a **blocked vein** meant that he had to have a vein graft to get the blood supply working again, but this became blocked and he lost a second toe owing to blood stagnation. At that time he was given kaltostat (a seaweed preparation). Twelve months later, a third toe started to go bad, as it was also blocked. He was given an angoplasty, and antibiotics, but they did not help him. After six months of this treatment, the toe showed no signs of improvement and it was developing **gangrene**.

At this point they were seeing a homoeopath, Elizabeth Oliver who suggested he try a Kombucha compress to try to save the third toe. Enid started brewing Kombucha at home and produced fine cultures. They drank the Kombucha tea, and one Saturday night Enid tried a Kombucha compress on John's toe which at that point was quite bad - discharging, smelly and showing bluey signs of gangrene. By the following Tuesday the pain had gone, and as she took off the compress, substantial healing had started. Unfortunately, the compress took off some skin as well. Next when she left on a compress for several days, and it dried up like brown paper, she soaked the foot and it came off easily. Finally she discovered that if she first soaked the Kombucha culture in water, it was kept moist on the foot and was more effective.

The nurse had been making regular visits to treat John's toe, by dressing it and giving reports to the general practitioner. The last time that the nurse saw him was in January 1997, and she was amazed at the healing in the toe, and said "Whatever it is you're doing, keep doing it! She said she would not come back unless he needed her.

Enid is impressed with the effectiveness of the Kombucha culture used as a poultice or compress. A neighbour's inflamed skin from an **in-growing toenail** healed very quickly. Enid and John's two year-old grandson had his **finger tip** almost **severed** by sharp metal. After binding some culture as a poultice, the finger tip completely healed.

Enid and John took Kombucha for only three months, and then gave up because of problems with their culture. They have now started up again after a six months gap, and she will see if it helps her oedema and John's diabetes. We'll tell you in the next printing how they get on. When we have a serious, long-standing condition we can't expect instant results. Nature works slowly, but surely!

ALAN & SHIRLEY BRITTON
are two people who work very intuitively with Kombucha. Both are in their late 40s. Alan is a musician who runs one of the leading New Country Music groups. Shirley has worked with animals all her life, and ran a successful animal shelter on holistic lines near Bristol for 15 years.

Alan was the one who contacted the Kombucha Network originally. In 1994 he saw an article in *Kindred Spirit* magazine, followed by a feature in *The Daily Mail*. He had a strong urge to get a book and to start brewing Kombucha. He insists that he knew from the start that Kombucha was something special.

Alan's lifestyle gave him high levels of **stress.** He has a **sensitive nervous system** which tends to produce a lot of **tension**. He felt sure that Kombucha would help him, and started drinking a wineglassful twice a day. At first, he felt dreadful and cut down the amount to a minimum. "First there were pains in my hips and legs, but in retrospect I think I was detoxifying too quickly. The oddest effect was memory loss and usually I have a very good memory. As a songwriter and performer I have to call up lyrics on stage every night, but during this time a hole would appear in my memory."

After two months he started to feel better, but kept on a low dose for another two months, being guided by how his body felt. He then gradually increased this again back up to two wineglasses a day. After two years, at the end of 1996, he felt he should stop, and didn't brew any Kombucha for six months. Then in the summer of 1997 he started again because he felt his body needed it. He was not on any medication at all during this time.

Alan says that Kombucha gives him more energy and helps him with his stress. He feels it cuts out the highs and the lows, and his nervous system feels more balanced. The word he uses is 'alignment'. For him Kombucha seemed to work first on the gut flora, and then on the nervous system. He says he gives the culture the honour and respect it is due.

Shirley, since the age of eleven years old, has been troubled with **arthritic hips, knees** and **hands**, usually showing as a painful swelling. For years she also suffered from **Irritable Bowel Syndrome**. In 1992 when her business collapsed and her father died, she developed more acute symptoms, for which the doctor prescribed painkillers, Ibroprofen and sleeping tablets; she had a bad reaction and stopped taking them. Her condition was diagnosed as **fibro-myalgia**, which is similar to M.E (Chronic Fatigue Syndrome), and also to arthritis. (Shirley, in fact, now believes that this is what she had been suffering from over the years, rather than arthritis.)

Like Alan, her initial reaction to Kombucha was a little unpleasant, with stiff and painful muscles and she reduced the dose down to one tablespoon of Kombucha a day. Shirley noticed almost at once that her bowel movements changed and became regular. She had assumed that it was quite normal for people to have constipation alternating with diarrhoea, so when this pattern stopped it and she became regular, she found it quite strange. As her symptoms eased, she increased the dose, after a month, to a tumblerful a day.

Shirley started training in Reiki. At this point she believes that her body was telling her that she had had enough Kombucha for the time being, and stopped taking it. She has never followed any other alternative therapies, except for Kombucha. Though she still goes to the doctor occasionally, it is without much enthusiasm as she feels that she hasn't had much help for her illnesses from orthodox medicine. Shirley feels she understands her own body much better now.

After Shirley and Alan had both had a break from Kombucha, they started to brew again successfully, using a culture that they had stored in their fridge for six months. Shirley says that, with a combination of regular exercise, her Reiki healing and a tumblerful of Kombucha first thing every day, she has never felt more alive. She feels that Kombucha has a special life force that helps build up her own.

Shirley has used her instinctive feelings about the healing power of Kombucha in combination with her natural affinity with animals and has helped a foal and a dog in remarkable ways. (*See* Chapter 14)

MICHAEL STRABANE

(aged 63) has been in three armies, and was for a time in business, and then became a civil servant. Like many people of his age, he had been a heavy smoker earlier in life (100 cigarettes a day). He gave up smoking and drinking about 15 years ago when he joined the Transcendental Meditation movement. In 1988 he had a **heart attack** caused by pressure in his business and has suffered from **angina** ever since. He used Nu-Seals aspirin 75mg and Nitrolingual spray for under the tongue is case of a bad attack. He has suffered from **asthma** since 1990 for which he used two inhalers (Becotide and Ventolin) and also took two Neulin SA 175mg daily.

Michael was prone to **hay fever** and was put on a nine-week course of injections in 1992. It turned out that he was allergic to the treatment, and suffered severe loss of energy, cramps in the feet and toes, a lack of sensation up to the knees and total disorientation. As an emergency, he saw a young woman doctor (who had just qualified) who mistook his symptoms for a psychotic seizure and had him committed to a psychiatric hospital, heavily sedated.

Later, coming round from the drug and realising where he was, Michael escaped to a local hospital where his daughter worked, and on examination was diagnosed as suffering from **diabetes**. After being prescribed various tablets, he found that a strict diet and the tablet Glucobay three times a day was best for him. So in total he was taking seven tablets and two inhalers daily.

In June 1997 Michael was given a Kombucha culture by an Indian friend and he started brewing right away. Within one month all his discomforts ceased and life became easier for him. He started with a wineglassful three times a day and, by the second month of drinking Kombucha, had given up all his medications.

He still has all the drugs in the medicine cupboard, but feels he no longer needs them. Michael had taken for granted that his digestion was irregular, so when it cleared up, this was an unexpected dividend. He says he wakes up in the morning feeling great, has bags of energy, his breathing is almost back to normal and he can do all the jobs around the garden that before taking Kombucha were really quite a strain.

Michael says he believes that Kombucha is a God-given help for many afflictions. He has introduced Kombucha to many friends since the restoration of his own good health. Many of them have reported significant relief since taking Kombucha. His **brother** started to drink Kombucha tea, and sometimes puts a pint of it in his bath which he finds very invigorating; at 67 years he is still able to do full handstands!

Michael's nephew suffers from **asthma** and needs to be propped up on five pillows to help him sleep. After taking one glass of Kombucha each night before going to bed, he felt relaxed and well enough to remove three of the pillows and slept all night for the first time in years. One of Michael's friends is a lady who was **stung** by a wasp; she put some of the Kombucha tea on the sting and the pain immediately disappeared. One man who was about to put down his dog which had a bad **skin disorder**, was persuaded to bathe it with Kombucha tea, and after several applications the disorder cleared up. Michael knows some racing greyhound owners who feed spare Kombucha cultures to their dogs.

Michael also dabs Kombucha tea on his face and lets it dry naturally, he feels his facial skin tightening.

After a couple of months of drinking Kombucha tea, Michael began brewing in a 26-pint Continuous Fermentation Jar, and has increased his consumption. He says he just loves Kombucha and feels like a 30-year old, and would love to see Kombucha therapy as part of normal preventative medicine. He also believes that a positive attitude will help the Kombucha therapy to better effect. Michael still meditates every day and uses a mind-lab machine to help with relaxation. He affirms that he is 125% in favour of Kombucha and is a great missionary for the brew in his community.

LOLO KRIKORIAN

(aged 53) has been taking Kombucha for 1½ years, with one break of three months. She is very enthusiastic about Kombucha with most of her family, including her daughter, mother and sisters, now using it too.

Lolo, the eldest of seven daughters, had never enjoyed the best of health. As a little girl she always complained of a tired feeling and pain in her muscles. She had **asthma** and a tendency towards **lung** and **throat infections**. After taking Kombucha tea for a period of time Lolo says her difficulty with breathing eased and she can now breathe more normally. She says also that she has much more energy now as a consequence.

Lolo also had a **stomach ulcer** from the age of 13. None of the medication she took seemed to help with the symptoms, and after only one week of taking Kombucha, she noticed a relief in the excess acidity.

As well as drinking Kombucha tea, Lolo puts it on her hair and swears by it. She had developed severe **eczema** on her scalp with balding patches and rapidly thinning hair which failed to respond to treatment with polytar shampoo. She experimented with Kombucha tea, pouring a glassful on her hair and leaving it for up to three hours. She did this daily for one week, also covering her hair with a plastic bag to help keep the moisture in. To her great surprise she found that her hair had stopped falling out, and the eczema was greatly improved. Within a few weeks, fine hair began to reappear on her bald patches and the new hair was growing back darker, giving, according to her daughter, the impression of 'highlights'. Today Lolo's eczema has completely gone on her head and she now uses normal shampoo - though she still uses Kombucha at least once a week, leaving it on for a minimum of 3-4 hours. At other times, she uses it as a rinse/conditioner. Her hair has continued to improve in texture and volume and the colour has continued to grow darker!

Lolo keeps a bottle of Kombucha in the bathroom at all times and uses it regularly as an astringent and toner which she claims makes her skin feel nourished. Another tip from Lolo is that she uses mature Kombucha - i.e. a brew that has been allowed to become nearly vinegar - and says it is very good on greasy hair.

Lolo has also used Kombucha soaked in a pad of cotton wool and dabbed it over some eczema patches on her cheeks, leaving it on overnight. Her facial eczema has cleared up and people have told her how much better her skin looks.

Arthritic pains which she had all over her body have also eased 3 months after beginning the Kombucha therapy. When she stopped taking Kombucha this year the pains came back with a vengeance .

Lolo, who used to be a (UK) 8-10 dress size, started taking Hormone Replacement Therapy and went up to a size 18. Even on a very strict diet she lost nothing in three months. While drinking Kombucha she has lost weight, reducing to a size 12. Her method is to drink a glassful at least an hour before breakfast, and well before all other meals. Lolo has a big family and is so enthusiastic about Kombucha that she is converting them all.

Daughter - (aged 20) has described three separate incidences when Kombucha proved beneficial. First, on returning, with a cold, from a pub with a smoky atmosphere, she used Kombucha as a soothing application to **sore and swollen eyes**. Secondly, she placed a piece of the fungus, dipped repeatedly into the liquid, on a stubborn **boil** under her arm. The pus was drawn out and the boil was well on the way to recovery the next day. Thirdly, on a hot day, the skin between her legs became chafed. She applied the Kombucha fungus as a poultice and, by the next morning, the **rash and soreness** had gone.

Lolo remembers that her friend's father was given Kombucha in a Russian hospital in Iran thirty years ago. Russian doctors, she says, frequently used to prescribe Kombucha therapy for liver and kidney patients.

ROB HALCRO

has suffered from severe **eczema** and **asthma** for most of his life. In addition he feels he has had to contend with the indignities of illness and dependence created by the treatments which were meant to help him. He says that he felt a disadvantage being born a sensitive child into a family that misunderstood and was intolerant of his condition. Rob's skin problem started before he was one year old.

From an early age Rob said that he had to take many medicines - drugs for everything. These included eye ointment (containing topical steroids) for **conjunctivitis**, Vallergan syrup for sedation, and Ephedrine tablets for **asthma**. Later he was put onto steroid inhalers and topical steroids (Dermovate).

In 1981 Rob left home and started working for the civil service. Within five years he says that the cocktail of medicines he was taking, as well as smoking cannabis, had so confused him that he suffered a succession of **mental and emotional breakdowns**, with further drug treatment for **depression**. He turned to psychotherapy treatment and yoga which helped wean him off soft drugs and alcohol. He had not realised, however, that it was his addiction to topical steroids that caused **dehydration, immune problems**, and massive **energy fluctuations**. By 1988 Rob was unemployed and on health disability financial support. He began a course of acupuncture and herbal treatments, healing and more psychotherapy. The last two, he believes, were the more efficacious for him. Though feeling in better balance physically, his personal life was in some turmoil.

In 1993 Rob had **kidney problems** which called for surgery - he found the major operation particularly traumatic. He was also taking hydrocortisone at this time for his eczema, still using a steroid inhaler for asthma, and now suffered **chronic indigestion** after the operation. Rob, who has remained a very sensitive person, believes that it took eight months for the morphine injected in hospital to leave his physical body and a further six months to leave his energy bodies, which he experienced like 'a shift in gears'

His ex-partner's daughter brought a Kombucha culture back from Australia in April 1996. Rob read about its ability to remove toxins and started taking small amounts of Kombucha tea. Soon he noticed an improvement in his energy level. Over the next eight months, his body went through a process of detoxification which he noticed in different areas of the body, from the sinus mucous, to the digestion and his bowels. He says: "It felt much like a gentle encounter that allowed me to comprehend bit by bit the process unfolding. At worst I felt as though I had a long drawn-out heavy cold. That's all! How did I know that Kombucha was working? By the confidence I gained to give up different medicines." The digestive medication was given up first (Tagamet 400mg once daily, and Motilium 10mg three times a day), then the pain killers for acute back muscle spasms (Dihydrocodeine 60mg twice daily) and Anusol ointment for haemorrhoids was replaced by homoeopathic Rescue Remedy Cream. Finally he gave up the hydrocortisone (Efcortelan 0·5%).

Rob's earlier brews of Kombucha tea were rather acid and he decided to take his Kombucha brewing in hand. He improved his utensils and switched to organic tea. He got three heating trays and found that if he took the brew off one day early and put it in a 5-litre demijohn with water valves, it would keep on a kitchen shelf for a couple of weeks, and improve in quality. If the brew does go acidic, he says, he adds it to his bath, $1^{1}/_{2}$ -litres/ (3-pints) at a time. He loves to do this because he feels that it gently enters his system and gives him an 'inside awareness' of his healing. He describes his healing process with Kombucha as "a subtle change which seems also to affect my thinking".

In 1996 Rob embarked on a dance degree course and found that, as a result, his sleep and eating habits have changed.

One of the most interesting insights Rob had was his discovery that he gained more improvement from Kombucha when he started caring more for himself and making it with a loving attitude, which included improving his brewing skills. He feels that the key to healing is very often to regain self love. He speaks of his Kombucha with affection as "a sensitive and almost 'conscious' entity which became a role model for me of unconditional love".

Rob has a strong sense of confidence that Kombucha has helped him a lot. All but a few occasional patches of eczema have gone completely. He feels that his body and blood have been cleaned up, and he is more balanced. He uses little topical steroids now. Rob says that it is important for him to listen to his body's needs and stops taking Kombucha for a period of time when he feels it is right to do so. He understands that taking Kombucha has allowed him to be more at ease with his own sensitivity and to be in touch with himself, to be able to choose; that it acts more at an energy level, which will then affect his physical. He gives away the Kombucha tea, but tends to hold onto his cultures, digging bits of them into his pot plants. "They love it", he insists!

It is often not easy for people to understand how Kombucha therapy works on a holistic level, as we are so used to thinking always about physical symptoms. We have included the story of Hugo, whose most distressing experience was to lose his **mind function**, and for whom Kombucha played a significant part in his rehabilitation.

HUGO HENDERSON

is the fourth of five children, whose parents' marriage broke up when he was eleven. He was in a London school where drugs were available, and he started smoking marijuana when he was thirteen. He admits that he tends to do things to excess, but that it was his active curiosity about analysing his mental state that drew him into deeper experimentation. Acid and ecstasy were the next drugs to experience when he was 14, and cocaine when he was 16.

Hugo left home when he was 17, and having a natural aptitude for languages and an urge to travel, took a trip to Thailand a year later and, with a companion, experienced heroin for several months. It was not long after his return from a subsequent stay in France that Hugo became aware that the ecstasy was causing problems for his **liver** and **kidneys** and that the cocaine was causing **heart palpitations**. He went to Southampton University for a year to study European Policy with French, but as he didn't connect very well with his language course, Hugo decided to go to Columbia and Venezuela.

Hugo was, at that time, particularly dependent on the buzz from any drug, cocaine was then the most available, and in retrospect he realises that it was this that damaged his mind function. He experienced memory loss, almost complete lack of connectedness in his thought patterns, and had what he thinks was a **nervous breakdown**. Accompanying this were acute **anxiety attacks**, breathing difficulties, heart pains, hot spots on the head and burning sensations on different part of his body. As a result of this breakdown, far from home, he was unable to help himself and suffered from severe malnutrition, and had the added problem of a jail sentence for stealing food in Venezuela.

By some miracle, Hugo managed to get home to Somerset, still in a shaky state and suffering anxiety attacks. Blood tests showed that both his liver and kidneys had inadequate function. He had **kidney stones**, pains up and down his body, and **inflammation**. After undergoing those tests at the Bath Association for Drug Rehabilitation, Hugo heard from them about Kombucha therapy. He started brewing Kombucha and drank a $^1/_3 ._1/_2$ wineglassful three times a day. He did not suffer any detoxification problems and, within a few days, felt a lot calmer. He says that as he felt energy moving through his body, it seemed to ease tension around the problem areas.

"This increase of chi energy gave me some kind of lift and a heightened sense of awareness - a feeling of being generally more in control psychologically. Two days after I ran out of Kombucha, I started to feel an increase in anxiety and tension again. There were no other factors which could have influenced this reversal."

Six weeks after Hugo started drinking Kombucha he had another blood test which showed that his liver and kidney functions were normal, for the first time in $2^1/_2$ years. He reports that his anxiety and tensions levels are now quite manageable, though he still has some abdominal pains. Returning to a caring home with good nutrition must have helped Hugo's rehabilitation, but he definitely feels that Kombucha therapy has contributed to a greater clarity of thought, a sense of greater awareness and better memory, as well as a sense of happiness and well-being.

While six weeks is not a long time to monitor the benefits of Kombucha therapy, the particular help it has given Hugo in that short time is encouraging, and we shall keep in touch with his progress. Perhaps one of the most interesting other reactions Hugo has had is that, within days of starting to drink Kombucha tea, he seemed to lose his **desire for alcohol**, even to the extent of being able to go into a pub (bar) without wanting a drink. At the time of writing, he still has no wish to return to alcohol, which, for over six years has been his main obsession.

CHAPTER 11

HEALTH, SELF-EMPOWERMENT AND NUTRITION, AN HOLISTIC VIEW

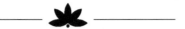

Whose Body is it Anyway?

There has never been a generation in modern times so much under threat from its own lifestyle. We may feel that our national priorities are wrong, or that technology has become a new religion. We may also feel powerless to influence the course of society, but we can at least have some control over our own life and, as a consequence, may come to recognise that we have more influence than we realise on the world around us. Most doctors are very caring and dedicated people. They are also trained to feel that they should be accepted as the ones who know what is best for *your* health. You are very fortunate if you have a doctor who will let you be involved in your own health decisions.

It is partly a generation problem. Older doctors often feel threatened by the idea of sharing their power with you. There is no question that we are likely to preserve our health for longer if we can find a doctor who is willing to empower us and discuss with us what our health needs are. It's our body, after all, and once we get in touch with it, with an open-minded and sympathetic doctor or practitioner to help guide and re-educate us towards good health, we are better equipped to face all that comes our way. In the end, after all, only we ourselves can really initiate a deep and lasting healing.

Energy Medicine

Contemporary science tends to believe that the physical world is all that there is. You may have observed how dismissive scientists can be when you talk about 'good vibrations', subtle energies, symbiosis, or even healing. 'New' medicine and 'new' science (though they are, in fact, based on ancient wisdom) now acknowledge that it is energy that influences the physical, or even creates it.[1] *Everything is energy*. The nursing profession knows this; Florence Nightingale's example still informs its traditions, and nurses know that compassionate care and a loving environment help patients to get better much faster. You probably know this from your own experience - that the quality of our energy affects our daily experience. When we feel centred, positive and clear, everything runs smoothly, food made with love tastes different, a positive, constructive attitude in a group discussion will result in a positive outcome, and so on. We are the creators of our own lives.

There is a fast growing interest in a branch of psychosomatic medicine called 'mind/body' medicine. This recognises the crucial part that attitude plays in one's health. The negative emotions that affect health mostly are fear, grief and resentment. Illness can bring such low energy and depression that we may not, for instance, feel that we have the motivation to do something like brewing Kombucha for ourselves, or the patience not to expect immediate results. Nature's way is slow but sure. The greatest support you can give to a sick parent, partner or friend is to help with their Kombucha brewing, give encouragement to persevere and the optimism for improvement which is often lacking in the one with the illness. Left to themselves, a sick person often wants quick relief, and will be drawn more to the promises of easy-to-swallow pills that may take away the pain, can suppress the symptoms, but certainly will not find the cause of the problem; indeed this approach frequently causes more problems! However, many who come to Kombucha therapy have already tried the quick fixes of drug cocktails that have not worked, and are looking for an alternative natural way.

Visualisation

Ernest Shattock was an admiral who, in his medical examination on retiring from the navy, was advised to have a hip replacement, necessitated by deterioration of bone and cartilage. He refused, and decided instead to take himself in hand. He realised that if he was to succeed he would have to learn how cell replacement works in the body, and focus his mind towards a reconstructive process. Knowing that the body's natural ability is to heal itself, he reasoned that he ought to be able to rebuild his disintegrating joint. His doctor provided all the necessary books on anatomy and physiology, and the encouragement to embark on a two-year programme of visualisation, in which he would be using a mind which he had trained over ten years in meditation practice. Alick got to know Shattock, and was so impressed by his integrity and his success, that he published two books about his experiences.[2]

While most of us probably cannot apply this degree of disciplined focus, we are all capable of bringing commitment to our own healing. We need to understand that all our other life outcomes depend on having a goal or vision of our future and then getting on with it. It is no good expecting or depending on other people to help us; our health depends on each of us taking personal responsibility and acting on it. It is rather like a golfer needing to visualise where the ball is to land for a really good shot.

Self-empowerment

By all means get advice from a health practitioner along the way, but make absolutely sure that you go to someone who will empower you. You might, for a start, find out if your doctor will actively encourage you to take part in making decisions about your own health. When it comes to assessing doctors, you should ask: What is their attitude towards medication? Do they look for the real cause behind illnesses? What do they think of complementary medicine, such as acupuncture or homoeopathy? Conventional medical thinking is sceptical because it does not have the science that can demonstrate how so-called alternative practices work. But when they do work, why knock them? The most precious of life's experiences, which are often the things we value most, cannot usually be 'explained' by scientific methods. Does that invalidate them? A holistically trained doctor or health practitioner is more likely to be able to help guide you towards an understanding of the cause of your illness. Only by doing this can real healing take place.

A friend told us about the library at the surgery he attends in a rural Somerset town. To quote from their leaflet, *A General Practice Patient's Library*: "The philosophy of the library is Empowerment, and thus 80% of the 300 titles lean toward complementary medicine, reflecting both the great thirst the general public has for the subject, and the limited capacity that books on disease have for empowering people. Initially most books purchased for the library were on disease rather than health, and borrowing was slow. The purchasing was changed to 'empowering health' rather than contemplating disease, and the borrowing rate has soared."[3]

Orthodox or Complementary?

This inevitably begs the question of whether to throw in one's lot with alternative medicine and forget about the conventional, allopathic form of medical treatment. Some people are convinced that complementary medicine can do everything and will stick exclusively to it. In many communities in the East, energy medicine is the traditional system and there is no question of using anyone other than a traditional acupuncturist or herbalist. However, most people in the West would feel uncomfortable about having nothing more to do with their orthodox doctor. Conventional medicine still does so much on a physical level to raise general standards of health, banish serious communal diseases and play an essential role in many life-threatening illnesses. We personally believe the best way forward lies in complementary medicine in which orthodox and alternative medicine each has its place and where both can work successfully together, if appropriate.

This is a view which is receiving much wider backing - not least from the Prince of Wales. In October 1997, Prince Charles made an impassioned plea for NHS patients to be given access to free complementary therapies. It is no secret that members of the royal family are great fans of complementary medicine, carrying homoeopathic remedies with them wherever they go and using the skills of doctors trained in various alternative techniques including acupuncture and osteopathy. Could this be the secret of the Queen Mother's amazing longevity and the Queen's continuing remarkably good health well into her seventies?

Prince Charles' words are worth repeating: "I am personally convinced that many people could benefit from complementary medicine.... We cannot afford to overlook or waste any knowledge, experience or wisdom from different traditions that could be brought to bear in the cause of helping those who suffer."

A Limited World View

The last 500 years (·00002% of human history) have seen a rapid expansion of the human rational (left brained) function, at the cost of our other abilities. Our culture is still hostage to deductive reasoning and rejects anecdotal experiences as 'unscientific'. There are intellectual power brokers at universities and medical colleges who have a vested interest in the status quo (i.e.

their theories) not being challenged. Nearly all advanced research is now dependent on subsidies from commercial interests, many of them connected with the chemical or drugs industries. Certainly research on new 'health' drugs is almost entirely funded by the multi-national drug companies who have a vested interest in their products being promoted and used by medical practitioners and hospitals.[4] It is worth considering how much profit is being made as a result of people's illnesses.

You can also understand the reluctance of health professionals to back something that supports general health and is free - and which might, consequently threaten their own jobs! It may sound cynical to say so, but many health organisations have a vested interest in people remaining ill. (This includes some charities and research projects as well as health professionals in all fields.) We need to ask why it is that certain people and organisations in our society seem to have a vested interest in people remaining sick. Could it have something to do with making money or holding on to power?

Lessons to Learn

Things are now beginning to change. There are some individual researchers (both young and old) who know that, unless the limited world view of human and planetary health shifts, the human species has a poor prognosis. They are showing how alienation from our own bodies and the envronment has produced a self-centredness which makes us short-sighted. The only antidote to this is to acknowledge, with humility, that we are a part of Nature. We can begin by looking at how Nature works and learn - from the experiences of BSE and the hazards of genetic manipulation, for instance - before we damage ourselves further. Sadly, the general trend in medicine, as in all the sciences, is still towards more and more specialisation which produces a narrow, exclusive, view.

Some of the media seem to feel under an obligation to take a sceptical view of anything which is not easily explained scientifically. In fact, they often have a 'specialist' on hand to give a 'balancing' or opposing view to complement what they consider to be unconventional. In talking about Kombucha on television we have been faced several times by an 'expert' with preconceived ideas and an apparent need to discredit it without ever having studied the existing research, or even tasted Kombucha tea. This produces an unbalanced and untruthful picture, and can make the viewer fearful without justification. This cynical type of journalism does not allow open and informed discussion of an ancient therapy which is used to great effect by scores of doctors and hospitals in Russia and further East. This policy seems immature at a time when it has never been more important to learn how to solve our problems cooperatively as mature adults.

Kombucha's Record

Kombucha therapy has a track record dating back more than 2,000 years. With the exception of a tiny number of cases of irresponsible misuse, it has done no-one any harm. On the contrary, it has helped millions of people, and never more so than today. It is true that modern orthodox medicine has also helped many millions of people and saved many lives, but its success is also tempered by its limitations. Thousands die every year from medical malpractice, or from the side effects of conventionally dispensed drugs. Sadly, medical politics rarely allow these statistics to be properly acknowledged or reported.

We have attempted in this book to lift the discussion about Kombucha therapy out of the level of 'fantastic claims' and place it in a setting where it can become better understood by those of a questioning mind. It is for this reason that we have included in-depth case histories only of people we have spoken to personally, and therefore whose authenticity we can confirm.

We are Killing the Earth

"This we know. The Earth does not belong to man; man belongs to the Earth. This we know.
All things are connected, like the blood which unites one family. All things are connected.
Whatever befalls the Earth befalls the sons of the Earth.
Man did not weave the web of life; he is merely a strand in it.
Whatever he does to the web, he does it to himself."[5]

The Earth is a living entity and, as with any organism, when something happens to one part of it, this has an affect on the whole. Pollutants are carried around by the circulation of the atmosphere and the oceans so that, for example, nuclear fallout from Chernobyl was found in the pristine wastes of Lapland and the Hebridean isle of Lewis. We are pouring wastes into the oceans, yet are surprised when we find fish stocks badly affected or dolphins dying. Human beings are also affected when the natural environment deteriorates. It is easier to understand physical pollution than energy pollution. The Earth's ecosystem is a highly complex form of interdependence, intimately affected by any reduction of natural forest cover, from desertification, monoculture, urbanisation, opencast mining and electro-magnetic pollution, to the more obvious physical pollutants of modern industry, such as toxic wastes and petrochemicals. The problems are exacerbated by the emergence of self-serving multinational or transnational organisations who have no interest in the health of the environment and are able to do exactly what they want, without accountability or regulation. Governments too can act with appalling self-interest, and will continue to act irresponsibly until we realise that things must change. We need to wake up, take a good look at what is going on in the world around us and say, "No more destruction and pollution!". We are killing both the natural world <u>and</u> ourselves.

Living Only for Myself

It amazes us that many nutritionists, scientists and medical experts don't seem to see that we are doing the same things to our own bodies, with similar disastrous consequences. We have little information on what happens to our bodies after prolonged misuse through consuming food - coloured, flavoured and sweetened with countless chemicals. We may think we are eating natural, healthy foods when we choose conventionally grown fruit and vegetables, little realising that they have usually been force-grown with chemicals below and above the ground, and even sprayed with more chemicals after picking in order artificially to preserve their cosmetic appearance and shelf life. Even water, the most common substance on Earth and in the human body, and a life-giver to both, is fast becoming irreparably poisoned. So-called 'purification' of our drinking water involves a cocktail of chemicals which are supposed to render it harmless. The oceans, air and land are becoming polluted, and so are our own bodies.

It is not hard to see that the Earth and our human bodies are not healthy and will continue to degenerate. This will contribute to the social sickness of our societies if we don't wake up and do something about it now. The breakdown is so serious that some informed environmentalists give us only 40 years before the Earth may become quite inhospitable to humanity.

Taking Responsibility

Personal health crises play a significant part in opening a door to your true life path, and taking responsibility for our own health is part of this. Very often when someone has a critical illness they may think about death; or the meaning of their own life. Illness can play a very creative part in self-healing, and can indeed become our own teacher. Small recurring imbalances are warnings that all is not well with us and our life. If we don't pay attention and make some improvements, these imbalances may worsen, sometimes even becoming life-threatening diseases.

Our imbalances or illnesses haven't just appeared. They have taken years to cultivate, or may have been inherited. It is therefore important to be patient (the true meaning of being a 'patient') and continue using Kombucha therapy as a way of life in combination with other improvements in our lifestyle. We need steadily to regain good health and strength (there's no quick fix), and then maintain it. We can begin by starting to take responsibility for our own health, seeking medical advice when we need to, but constantly reminding ourselves, 'This is my own body and this is my world. If I don't take that responsibility, someone else might, and it could be to my detriment'.

Drinking Kombucha is a great way to begin. One of its main qualities is as a detoxifier, so it can start to cleanse an often over-stressed and polluted body. It strengthens the vulnerable immune system and organs, leading to improved body functioning and, as a consequence, to a better quality of life. Everyone knows that good health is the most important precondition for a good life, so take charge and start today - and thus help the health of the world tomorrow.

The Holistic View

The modern concept, that physicians must fight disease rather than cooperate with Nature to eliminate it, has divided medicine into two fields, allopathic and naturopathic. The philosophy of the natural health practitioner centres on the study of holistic health - that is, the whole of a person, mind and body and how to assist self-healing, rather than the study of disease and how to suppress it. Holistic health practitioners regard the suppressing of symptoms as futile, because the real cause of the illness has not been found. Suppressing symptoms in a sick body which is trying to heal itself is a sticking plaster approach which will do nothing to prevent the illness and symptoms recurring. It is important also to find out what you have been doing to have created the illness in the first place.

The body and mind are an integrated whole. While the allopathic doctor admits that Nature does heal, the holistic practitioner treats this fact as a natural law to be worked with, not flouted. An increasing number of allo-pathically-trained doctors are beginning to think holistically, usually in spite of their training. Some doctors are training in therapies such as homoeopa-thy and acupuncture on short courses that last only six weeks. A fully qualified homoeopath or acupuncturist takes 3 - 4 years to train, undergo-ing personal development as part of learning the true meaning of 'holism'. An allopathic doctor who can take a short course in those disciplines is not likely to learn more than a symptomatic use of remedies, and will not be equipped to practise holistically, have the time, or begin to understand how to get to the heart of the patient's problem and find the underlying cause, which is sometimes buried quite deep.

Natural medicine cooperates with the body's own healing forces by us-ing natural healing methods and assisting the cleansing and elimination processes of the body. There is no drug that will restore cell normality when malfunction has arisen from disease; this can only be achieved by estab-lishing normal metabolism in the body with the help of Nature.

Homeostasis = Healthful Equilibrium

When the body is functioning optimally, we are in a state of homeostasis. This means that all the internal systems of our body are in equilibrium, de-spite any variations in external factors. Homeostasis is maintained by the body's self-regulating and self-repairing ability, but, for these to function correctly, our diet and lifestyle must be balanced and supportive. If they are not, the correct balance of essential nutrients like enzymes and antioxidants, vitamins and minerals necessary for the maintenance of these functions and the protection of the body against harmful wastes, and their elimination will be disrupted. When homeostasis is disturbed, disease results. This begins within individual cells that, in turn, make up specific tissues and organs. When a cell's normal regulating and communication processes are altered, disease begins. The miracle of Nature is that all these processes are self-correcting when given a chance. This is what healing is about. The healing process can be assisted in many ways, but chemical invasion is not the way to do it, except in extreme illness when we have allowed the disease in our bodies to go too far.

The Mind-Body Connection

How then, do we apply these principles to Kombucha therapy? Kombucha affects the whole body rather than the symptomatic reactions to an illness. This means that it acts homeostatically by bringing different parts of the system into balance. The ideas we have about ourselves actually affect how our body responds. It is important, therefore, not to become obsessed with having our specific symptom relieved or suppressed, or for our disease to disappear, but to view that wish in a detached way.

We need to practise seeing ourselves as a whole body, not just as a dis-ease. If we do not feel well, it is good to think of ourselves only as being out of balance, and then to visualise coming back into balance; to have confidence that we have within us all that we need to become healthy. It's not so much a vague kind of faith healing as a very positive and constructive attitude that we give ourselves permission, that we have a 'right' to be well.[6] It is, in fact, what the body is always trying to do - heal itself; we just need to assist the process along and not block it.

Life's Turning Points

We can often look back on a particularly traumatic experience and realise that it was like a kick up the backside which helped to get us out of a rut. Objectively, these are the big learning experiences of life that build character and put us back on a challenging path that begins again to look like 'a journey'. At times it may be difficult to be positive about a traumatic event and it may then be wise to seek out a good counsellor who can help us see the wider horizons.

Emotions such as prolonged depression, sadness, anger or grief will eventually affect our body functioning, no matter how deep we bury or try to ignore them. We have to try to understand the cause of these feelings, and release them. It is well-known that a high level of stress can contribute to many illnesses and can destroy lives if it is allowed to. So, knowing that good health is the most important thing in life, it is vital to take heed and change.

Attitude is All-Important

Just as in self-hypnosis, an idea (usually positive), can be presented to the subconscious in order to bring about a change in pattern or attitude, so negative emotions and thoughts can be reinforced by constantly repeating inner expressions of self-doubt, such as, 'I am not good enough. I resent my job. I hate my life. I can't change'. Seeing how the mind-body connection works in our lives is an essential part of self-empowerment. We can begin to educate and change old life-patterns through our thoughts, breaking down our former set style of being and opening the door towards a growing, ever-changing creative new you. You are what you think, so think positively and it will change your life![7]

Empowering your Fungus

We both feel that Kombucha is a gift of Nature; that it has become widely available now because we need it more than we have ever done. Our immune systems are generally quite depleted because of inadequate nutrition, various forms of pollution (most of which we are completely unaware of), stress and fear of an uncertain future. We feel that treating our Kombucha culture with respect will empower it and ourselves even more. It may be for this reason that the communities in rural Russia that used Kombucha considered its cultivation and drinking it to be a sacred ritual.[8]

It is interesting to note here that laboratory tests have shown many times that water that has been 'treated' by a healer has a higher vitality than a control sample which has not. Don't forget that the Kombucha culture is alive and will respond to tender, loving care, just like any 'plant' or person will.

Beginning to Change

Maybe it will not be our arthritis that will be helped, it may be the digestion, or energy level. Coming into balance is a very individual experience. In association with Kombucha therapy, while our body is beginning to regain health and strength, it is a good opportunity for us to look at other aspects of our life that may have caused us to become out of balance or ill in the first place. It may be that our lifestyle or self-image needs to change before a real healing can take place. Some of us may be too self-centred, and need objective feedback on how we come across to others. Some of us may need to learn how to share our problems as part of the healing process.

Most of us are quite out of touch with our bodies and need to learn to listen more to what they can tell us about our imbalance. Perhaps we are always trying to escape through outside stimulation, noise, music and chatter instead of just listening to what is really going on inside ourselves. We may not like it at first, but if we have no awareness of our own processes, how can we make changes? Giving attention to our body is not as hard as we may think; we just have to be open to the idea of it telling us what it needs.

Lessons - How Anyone can be Your Teacher

Mari would like to share two experiences of how she was helped by very special people to accept herself more honestly and find deep healing:

"Twelve years ago I began to go to Tai Chi classes (meditation in movement). The centredness of the movement and the silence became a mirror, and I began to see myself as I really was. I saw myself as needing to be good, to be right and wanting attention. I didn't like what I saw. It made me feel insecure and, after the first few classes I would go home in tears. After a few weeks, we began as students to share with each other and with the teacher what we were experiencing. We could see our imperfections and many of us started the process of acceptance of who we really are, which initiated the change and real healing in our lives. It wasn't that scary either."

"The second experience was when I was recently worried about heart palpitations caused by too much stress. Alick recommended I have a checkup with a particular doctor whom he liked, in the local practice, as I hadn't seen one for years. This doctor did not write a prescription to calm me down (which I would have thrown away anyway). Instead, he helped me with his guiding and searching conversation and presence - empowering me to find the cause behind my problem. I am myself a health practitioner who reminds and helps clients to get balance back into their lives. But we often forget what we know, and this quiet doctor reminded me to make the changes myself that would help my health. He helped me to find the real cause deeply buried behind the presented cause and symptoms and to remember what really makes my heart sing and be happy. He was, indeed a true healer and he gave me the time and space to explore. We learn, forget, and then remember again and again what is right for us. We have to remind each other to be kind and show ourselves compassion."

A wise teacher once described human nature as being essentially perfect, like the sun, shining bright, clear, strong and beautiful, dulled only by the clouds that we have created for ourselves in our life.

It's never too late to explore some new way of developing awareness in our lives. There are now lots of courses and experiential workshops to go to, such as yoga, tai chi, meditation, massage, artistic activities and movement. Our health is also dependent on regular exercise. By keeping the blood and the muscles well oxygenated we avoid the energy blocks that make us feel apathetic and uninspired.

The Importance of Nutrition

At the heart of our health problems today lie very poor standards of nutrition, driven by a multinational food industry which has little interest in real nutritional values. The more food manufacturers try to imitate natural flavours in their products, the more profit they make. The adulteration of processed food and the addition of chemicals have unknown consequences for our long-term health. New technologies, like those producing genetically engineered soya beans or tomatoes, should be a red flag, warning us that it is time to make our own decisions about our diet, because we know "we are what we eat". We must demand accurate food labelling and realise that only natural food is good for us - it is common sense really.

We also need to learn what constitutes a balanced diet.[9] Heart disease is the biggest killer today in most European countries and in the USA. The current wisdom on its prevention is to have five portions a day of fruit or vegetables (preferably organically grown), to avoid smoking and to take regular exercise. This may sound simplistic, but it makes sense. The next biggest killer is cancer, and this is at the centre of immune deficiency problems where high toxic levels caused by chemical additives, smoking and pollution are the culprits (Kombucha can help here). Stress and many more complex problems brought about by unhealthy and unhappy lifestyles are also often indicated as causes.

The Digestion

The digestive system is perhaps the most personal part of the body, in the sense that for each of us it is tuned slightly different. That is why we have to become more aware of what we individually need in order to keep our digestive system in balance. There are some general guidelines: for most of us a diet lacking in fresh vegetables and fruits but high in fat and sugar, fried and processed foods, tea, coffee and alcohol is not healthy. These are predominantly acid-forming foods, and an over-acid environment can eventually enter our bloodstream. However, it has to be acknowledged that lifestyle plays as important a part as nutrition. Too much stress, in whatever area of your life, combined with unsatisfactory dietary habits, can bring about illness. Most Western people exercise too little. Regular exercise can do wonders for over-acidity, poor metabolism and blocked energies.

Microwave Cooking

Recent research suggests that cooking or heating food in microwave ovens can cause molecular damage which, when eaten, can lead to abnormal changes in human blood. These changes can cause deterioration of the immune system. In a small, but well-controlled trial, eight people were given either normally cooked or microwaved food over a few days. Blood samples were taken before and at several intervals after meals. Whereas the blood samples of the people eating normally cooked food showed little change, the blood of the people who had eaten microwaved food showed a drop in lymphocytes, the white blood cells critical to immune health.[10]

What to Do About it

People usually complain about the higher cost of fresh organic food. In fact many people don't even add up the weekly cost of the fast foods or the precooked convenience foods that have become so popular. A comparison of the total may show that you can well afford to pay a bit more for organic food that is really so much better for your health. As the demand for organic food increases, its price will come down. If the price of the mass-produced, chemically grown food included its hidden costs - the damage to ecosystems caused by chemicals in the soil and the 'food miles' involved in the enormous distances the food is usually transported, it would be a lot higher. The answer is simple - eat fresh and locally grown food and support the local economy. The big supermarkets have been surprised at the demand for their organic produce and are trying to encourage more organic growing in Britain which has the smallest area in Europe under organic cultivation. They are even beginning to sell local produce as a special attraction. Could this be coming full circle?

There are now many wholefood sources, so you could look in your area for one. In our Somerset village, we are a group of local families who put in a weekly collective order to our local organic farm who make fresh vegetables, organic meat and other produce available to subscribers, thereby cutting out the middle person. Many parts of the country have similar 'box' schemes. The lesson is that it is advantageous to cooperate in local group buying, as it builds up community spirit and support. The produce is also very fresh and usually cheaper than in the supermarket

Disease and the Environment

There are debilities like Chronic Fatigue Syndrome and Multiple Sclerosis which are little understood and are becoming more widespread, even among the young. Arthritis and Alzheimer's Disease have always been with us, but they seem to affect a wider range of the population now, showing more in younger people than in the past. There are many new viral conditions and a worrying emergence of diseases that are resistant to overused antibiotics. Often directly connected to our polluted environment are the increasing numbers of children with eczema, asthma and chronic allergies. These are caused by immune function deficiency and can therefore be helped by Kombucha therapy.

Each person has his/her own weakness which shows at times of stress and imbalanced life-style. It may be the stomach, liver, skin, heart or lungs. Whenever we don't look after ourselves our weakness will show itself. Through awareness we can begin to look after our weaknesses and learn to change our ways through them. We can all be surprised how many possibilities for a wider healing can emerge when the truly holistic view is taken of our health and of the wider environment.

Genetic Engineering

One of the big issues that has electrified opinion in every country in the world is that of genetic engineering. Scientists have pioneered these new technologies (not always with the best intentions), for 'improving' the capabilities of plants or correcting the genetic errors responsible for human disease. However, there are real and justifiable fears that the presence of foreign genetic elements might adversely affect the normal functions of cells.[11] In addition, as long as the subtle or non-physical aspects of the human being are not taken into account there is risk of making terrible and irreparable mistakes.[12] The reasoning that the scientists are giving to support genetic enginering is that it makes environmental sense as less fertilisers and pesticides will be needed on the crops. This is rubbish! Chemicals were never needed in the first place. Plants, in healthy soil, can resist most bugs. It is chemicals poured onto the land that have killed the vital bacteria, rendering the soil lifeless, which then creates a demand for even more fertilisers ... and so on. The land is becoming a desert, and the only way forward is to rediscover Nature's balance, working with, rather than against her.

Inherited Defects

The rapid development of genetic science has also led to greater awareness of weaknesses that we may have inherited from our parents and further back. Many families still carry echoes of the serious communal diseases that were rampant two or three centuries ago, like diphtheria, cholera, tuberculosis and syphilis. You may insist that modern medicine has banished them, but in energy terms they can still affect us. Through our DNA we carry the code of our forebears. These inherited defects can be treated homoeopathically (there is a new specialisation in homoeopathy called psionic medicine that does this).[13] Another way to look at the problem is the more psychological/spiritual view of 'healing the family tree'.[14] When we become truly aware of our life path and have a real sense of 'why we are here', we can then consciously exorcise these 'ghosts' of the past and, in a sense, come to terms with and heal our own and our whole family's weaknesses. Our modern society has forgotten the importance of families in the human evolutionary journey. It is common for many people to become aware of this when they are dying, when a natural urge to 'put things right' and heal a wounded relationship suddenly overtakes them.

DNA Balancing

Viktor Schauberger, an Austrian scientist, demonstrated that the creative basis of all life is the non-physical or energy level.[15] This, for example, is how we can influence matter or events with our minds. Energy medicine works on this basis, which is why it can be so effective, particularly with causative factors. DNA contains the genetic instructions for all living organisms. Science has only been concerned with the physical aspects of the genetic code, yet it undoubtedly has a non-physical component. Some researchers have suggested it is possible that Kombucha might also work at the subtle level of

DNA and energy balancing. At a time when so much change is taking place in our world couldn't this only be for the good?

In Summary

It is much better not to wait till your deathbed to forgive others or to recognise the purpose of your life. Here and now is the only place to begin, because the only way we can heal the world and our family is to begin with ourselves. The holistic view of self-healing begins with our own bodies. It can expand as far as we want to take it, and beyond. Each moment of every day is a new beginning. Let us all start today with the first step towards self-empowerment, self realisation, good health and happiness. The world will change for the better as a consequence.

Living by the Laws of Nature

The naturopath Robin Needes gives the following guidelines to 'Living by the laws of Nature':[16]

"This involves living in such a manner that the optimum health of the organism (the body) is maintained. The fundamental requirements are:
- a clean environment externally and internally - which means clean air, water and food, as well as attention being paid to the function of all the body's elimination channels.
- sunshine and fresh air, and living in a temperature zone for which the body was designed.
- adequate rest, sleep, exercise and attention to personal hygiene.
- whole foods with no additives, eaten in a pleasant environment and to the point of adequacy only.
- a healthy, relaxed state of mind and a correct mental attitude to life - positive, creative, constructive and relaxed."

We end on a note of healthy irreverence by Walt Whitman:
"This is what you should do: love the Earth and Sun and the animals, despise riches, give alms to everyone who asks, stand up for the stupid and the crazy, devote your income and labour to others, hate tyrants, argue not concerning God, have patience and indulgence toward the people, take off your hat to nothing known or unknown or to any man or number of men, re-examine all you have been told at school or church or in any book, dismiss what insults your own soul, and your very flesh shall be a great poem."

REFERENCES

1   Energy Medicine ref.

2   Shattock, Ernest, *Mind Your Body: A Practical Method of Self-Healing*: Turnstone, 1979; *A Manual of Self-Healing* : Turnstone, 1982

3   From a leaflet describing "A General Practice Patient's Library" at the Springmead Surgery, Chard, Somerset.

4   The British New Labour Government has named 18 drug companies (including the best known) that have been offering bribes to doctors to use their products, and plan to crack down on this common practice: *The Observer*, 27 Jul.97.

5   Chief Seattle (1786-1866)

6   Shapiro, Debbie, *Your Body Speaks Your Mind:* Piatkus, 1995

7   Hay, Louise, *You Can Heal Your Life:* Eden Grove, 1987.

8   Frank, Günther, *Kombucha: Healthy Beverage and Natural Remedy from the Far East:* Ennsthaler, 1991.

9   Davies, Jill, *Self-Heal: Pathfinder for Herbalism and Natural Healing* : Gateway, 1998.

10 Valentine, Tom, "Hidden Hazards of Microwave Cooking": *Nexus New Times*, vol.2, No.25 Apr.1995.

11 Ho, Dr Mae-Wan, *Genetic Engineering - Dream or Nightmare?:* Gateway, 1998.

12 Coudris, René, *The Roswell Message:* Gateway, 1997.

13 Upton, Carl, *Psionic Medicine,* Routledge, 1974 & Element, 1983.

14 McAll, Dr Kenneth, *Healing the Family Tree:* Sheldon, 1982.

15 Coats, Callum, *Living Energies: Victor Schauberger's Brilliant Work with Natural Energies Explained:* Gateway, 1996.

16 Needes, Robin, *You Don't Have to Feel Unwell!: Nutrition, Lifestyle, Herbs and Homoeopathy - a Home Guide:* Gateway, 1994.

CHAPTER 12

LACTIC ACID FERMENTATION
& THE IMPORTANCE OF VINEGAR

Fermented Foods

There are several ways of keeping fresh food from going bad. The modern way is to add a preservative, which is usually in a chemical and not particularly healthy form. The ancient way was to use vinegar, lactic acid (usually from sour milk) or lemon juice. But the best way of all is fermentation, a process which produces naturally the substances which will preserve it. In addition, fermentation can improve the taste, and make fats and proteins in the food easier to digest. It also helps to create an environment which discourages pathogenic organisms (*See* "Probiotics", p.14). That is why Kombucha tea, a lactic acid fermented food drink, is so good for the digestive system.

Primitive peoples all over the world developed foods fermented with lactic acid. They relied on these to promote their health and vitality well into old age. The fermented foods popular in the Mediterranean countries included sauerkraut, pickles, yogurt, kumiss, olives, buttermilk, kefir, wine and beer. In Asia they included tempeh, kimchee, sauces like soy and tamari, sake and beer.

Fermentation goes on naturally in certain plants and fruits which contain sufficient sugars, such as grapes, cucumbers, beetroot, cabbage. Lactic acid in the silage process prevents stored grass and grains from rotting. Milk ferments easily to make products like yogurt, kumiss and kwass. The same process is at work with sourdough bread, preventing it from going bad.

The Value of Lactic Acid

The health of indigenous peoples who used fermented foods in their regular diet has been well established by research.[1] Dental decay and degenerative conditions, such as heart disease, arteriosclerosis, arthritis and diabetes were very rare. Acetic acid which is used today as a food preservative has neither the nutritive nor probiotic qualities of lactic acid, though it does possess healing qualities of its own (see below).

Because Kombucha produces a significant amount of lactic acid in addition to many other valuable nutritients, it is superior to fermented foods to which the lactic acid is added. (*See* p.15)

What is Vinegar?

Kombucha's history is inevitably shared with one of man's oldest foods, vinegar. Vinegar is 5% acetic acid, which is what gives the characteristically sour taste to vinegar. Acetic acid is one of the major organic acids produced in Kombucha tea. The acetous fermentation which creates the acetic acid is due to a tiny micro-organism, the vinegar bacillus, a bacterium which is present everywhere in the atmosphere, which is why the early vinegar producers were so successful. There are different species of these bacteria which digest the alcohol and convert it to organic acids, by the fermentation process.

Vinegar and Fermentation

The sugar added to Kombucha tea in its warm environment is first converted to alcohol by yeasts in the Kombucha culture. The alcohol is almost completely changed into acetic acid by bacteria which thrive on B vitamins produced by the yeast. It is this which gives Kombucha its sweet-and-sour smell of fermenting apple cider. The longer the fermentation process goes on, the greater amount of acetic acid is produced. After a couple of weeks in the recommended temperature, the Kombucha tea will be too sour to drink, but the vinegar produced is excellent. In fact the qualities of Kombucha vinegar are superior to those of apple cider vinegar, popularised by Dr. Jarvis in his *Vermont Folk Medicine*.[2] What the apple variety will do, Kombucha vinegar will also, and more, because of the way its particular constituents come together. (*See* Chapter 3, "How Does the Fungus Work?")

The History of Vinegar

The oldest form of vinegar, that associated with wine or beer that has 'gone off' with age, or has been intentionally put through a second fermentation, has been in use for at least 10,000 years. The origin of the word is from the French 'vin aigre' (sour wine). The Babylonians used to make wine from dates. About 4,000 years ago it had become widely used and highly regarded as a flavouring for food, especially with the addition of spices such as saffron, garlic and tarragon, which enhanced its qualities for food preservation.

The Assyrians, Greeks and Romans regarded vinegar as an important medicine, in addition to its preservative value, in flavouring certain foods. They understood that it helped digestion, liver and gallbladder functions and prevented scurvy. Hippocrates (490-425BC) developed the use of vinegar into a fine science. He mixed it with honey to make 'oxymel' to which was attributed a large range of cures for acute illness, especially in the digestive system and the kidneys. Dr Jarvis also says that honey, when mixed in, enhances the effect of apple cider vinegar.

The Jews valued vinegar highly for flavouring and preserving food, as a medicine and even as a drink. It is mentioned many times in the Bible. The Romans introduced vinegar into Britain. They used it for dressing wounds and infectious sores. 'Thieves vinegar' got its name during the Great Plague, when some enterprising robbers used vinegar to protect themselves from contamination while they robbed the homes of plague victims.

Vinegar is said to have saved thousands of lives during the US Civil War and in the Crimean and Boer Wars when it was used as a disinfectant. It was also widely used since ancient times as a household cleanser.

Modern Uses of Vinegar

Today vinegar is still mainly used in connection with food, widely employed as a food preservative, taste improver, and meat tenderiser. Its value as a disinfectant is being rediscovered; recently someone had the idea of using vinegar in the prestigious Yale-New Haven hospital in the US. It was found to be more effective than commercial disinfectants in sterilising operating-room surfaces.[3]

The American determination to synthesise everything has resulted in commercial distilled malt vinegar now being permitted to be made from petroleum sources. So be careful before you use American malt vinegar for food preparation!

While the use of vinegar for healing purposes has largely been forgotten in the West, in Japan it is still an old favourite. Commercial vinegar is made from the leftovers of rice wine (sake) made from bleached rice. The Food Research Laboratories in Tokyo have found that vinegar made directly from brown rice has five times the amount of amino acids and organic acids than the commercial vinegar. Dr Yoshio Takino of Shizuka University has found that this vinegar helps to maintain good health and to slow down aging by helping to prevent the formation of two fatty peroxides. It also discourages free radicals and inhibits cholesterol build-up in blood vessels.

Where does Vinegar come from?

Vinegar is the product of a natural process called 'acetous fermentation', which is the breakdown of alcohol when it comes in contact with oxygen. Most carbohydrates contain sugars, which on degeneration produce vinegar. The most familar of these are fruits, hops, rice and other grains. The vinegars best known are those from apples, and from any kind of wine which has been left to ferment beyond the drinking stage.

Kombucha tea is quite unlike any other fermentation process in that it does not depend on going through an alcohol stage. Because the sugar required for fermentation is added as free sugar, the acetic acid can be produced with only an insignificant amount of alcohol. The Kombucha culture floats on top of the brew so that it can get the oxygen it needs for the fermentation process. A vinegar will possess the basic nature and essential ingredients of the original food from which it came; in addition it contains generous amounts of health-promoting vitamins, enzymes, amino acids and trace elements.

Vinegars intended for industrial use are often distilled, through which they lose most of their therapeutic properties, and become the basic acetic acid. 'Mother of vinegar' is a term used to describe the mass of sticky scum which is formed by the beneficial bacteria on top of cider when alcohol turns into vinegar. This is often used by vinegar makers as a starter for new vinegars, and it was said to be endowed with nspecial healing properties. Basically this mother of vinegar is only a scum; it is a by-product which is not essential to the making of vinegar and is not to be confused with the Kombucha 'mother' culture. The Kombucha culture is a very much more complex organism; it is a cellulose pancake which is a symbiotic community of bacteria and yeasts which reproduce by binary fission.

Apart from the range of organic acids found in Kombucha which are more complex than those in apple cider vinegar, its advantage is that it only requires one longer fermentation. Kombucha vinegar is very useful for First Aid applications, food preserving, in cooking, the home, and any purpose that you would use for ordinary vinegar. (*See* Chapter 13 "Kombucha Recipes and Other Uses - Kitchen, Beauty and the Home" - which includes how to make and use Kombucha vinegar.)

REFERENCES

1   Price, Weston, DDS, *Nutrition and Physical Degeneration*: Price-Pottenger Nutrition Foundation, 1939: Keats Pubs, 1989.

2   Jarvis, Dr D.C., *Folk Medicine: A Doctor's Guide to Good Health*: W.H.Allen, 1960 & Pan, 1961.

3   *The Vinegar Book.*

KOMBUCHA RECIPES AND OTHER USES - KITCHEN, BEAUTY AND THE HOME

Kombucha's applications are wide and varied. In Chapter 7 ("A-Z") and in Chapter 8 ("First Aid") we have explained its wonderful healing properties for health purposes, but it doesn't stop here. Where Kombucha tea has been shown to be a very nutritious health 'food' drink it can be used in many food recipes too. Try Kombucha vinegar, which, like Kombucha tea, is also 'live' and will take you into another realm, enhancing your recipes. It is, of course, also far superior to any refined and processed vinegar, which has really no health value at all.

What can be healed inside the body with Kombucha can be repeated on the surface, helping to make our skin, hair and body beautiful. And in the home, vinegar has been used through the ages in all manner of ways; as a natural antiseptic, for removing limescale and cutting through grease and grime.

If we look carefully at the properties of Kombucha, we can become aware of the many, many ways in which it can be used in wise and natural applications, taking care of us throughout our lives. So let's not be slaves to consumption or respond to advertising by being told what we should have and need to buy. Let us all think again and look at what nature has given to us freely. Kombucha **is** a gift of Nature. It is economical and ecological, healing our bodies and our homes.

KOMBUCHA FOOD RECIPES

There are many interesting ways of using Kombucha tea and vinegar in recipes, not only in traditional fermented foods such as sauerkraut, but also in some more unusual and varied forms of food preparation such as: fresh fruity Kombucha drinks, home made bread and fruit tea cake, soups, sauces, salads and pickles, chutneys and some of the most delicious herb and fruit-flavoured vinegars.

We accept that in all forms of cooking natural foods we will destroy a certain amount of its nutritious value, and that most natural foods are better for us in the 'live', raw and vibrant state. Kombucha tea is no exception, when we are taking it in its natural and highly energetic healing form.

A diet with a high percentage of uncooked foods will have many health-promoting benefits which can include reversal of degeneration and long-term illness (*See* Leslie Kenton's books *Raw Energy* and *The Biogenic Diet*). However, while we believe that a large proportion of our daily intake should be fresh, organic and 'alive', we also need a whole range of other foods which will provide added nutrition, with different methods of preparation; steaming, baking, boiling etc. and according to season which gives balance and interest to our daily diet.

Kombucha becomes more intriguing when we increase our knowledge of it and we are constantly finding new and interesting ways of using it in food preparation. Many people remark to us how they too have noticed an interesting quality and taste in both fresh and cooked Kombucha dishes, and that there is another 'energy essence' to it, which is independent of any other ingredient.

We have given a few tried and tested recipes here for you to try, but they serve mainly to give you ideas on how to use Kombucha more widely in your own kitchen. Be adventurous, like the people who created them, and let us know what your successes are so that we all can share in the sheer delight, health and ever-growing fascination of Kombucha.

BAKING

Have a go at baking using Kombucha tea, feel and taste the difference with these two recipes!

LUCY'S KOMBUCHA TEA FRUIT TEA-CAKE

This recipe is very simple to make and is absolutely delicious. Try keeping it for a week to mature. Lovely spread with a little butter too.

Mix together:

- 350-gms/ 12-ozs (US: 1½-cups) mixed dried fruit
- 110-gms/4-ozs (US: ½-cup) dark brown sugar
- 150-mls/¼-pint (US: a little over ½-cup) Kombucha tea

Soak overnight and the next day add 1 beaten egg and ½-lb self-raising flour. Bake 1 hour 350°C/gas mark 4.

KOMBUCHA BREAD

You can use Kombucha tea in any bread recipe, but don't replace all the water with it. Instead use ½-Kombucha tea and ½-water. You will find that the bread dough is much creamier, and the baked bread has a very interesting flavour quite unlike any other. The crust is crisper and therefore makes lovely crisp bread too. Here is our bread recipe. It only has one proving, for us busy bees, and makes 3 very fine loaves. Can be frozen.

Ingredients:

- 1.35-kg/3-lbs (US: 11-cups) wholewheat flour
- 2 teaspoons salt
- 3 teaspoons dark brown sugar, honey or molasses
- 3 level teaspoons dried yeast
- 1-litre/2-pints (US: 5-cups) water (blood heat)

Method

Warm the flour and mix in the salt. Mix yeast with 3 tablespoons of warm water and

leave for 2 minutes. Add the sugar and leave a further 10-15 minutes. Pour into flour and add the rest of the water.

Mix well until elastic, and leaves sides of the bowl clean (this helps to form a well built loaf).

Divide dough, which should be slippery but not wet, into 3 x 2-pint (US: 2½-pints) tins, warmed and greased. Place in a warm place covered with a cloth and leave for 20 minutes or so until within ½-inch of the top of the tin.

Bake in a fairly hot oven, 400°C-Gas mark 6, for approximately 35-40 minutes.

FRUITY KOMBUCHA DRINKS

We have used both dried and fresh fruits in making Kombucha tea and drinks, and while we love Kombucha tea in its natural form, it is also nice to have a variety of recipes up our sleeves for added interest and fun for all ages.

Addition of Ginger and Lemon

The simplest way to add another flavour to your Kombucha tea is to add a slice or two of root ginger to the ferment for a nice wintry drink, or add a wedge of lemon to give it an extra refreshing zest.

FRUIT-FLAVOURED KOMBUCHA TEA

Many people have discovered the new world of Kombucha fruit tea by adding dried fruits, either loose or in tea-bag form, but please note that they should be *in addition to your tea*, green or black (as in the Batch Brewing and Continuous Fermentation methods). **Do not use them on their own** as this would affect the overall health and quality of the fungus and of the Kombucha tea.

Add 1-4 teaspoons or tea bags of dried fruit tea to green or black tea as in the Batch Brewing Method (*see* p.32). We use green tea and dried fruit tea in proportion 2:2, but some people like it stronger and use it in 2:4, especially for children or even 4:4. See how you like it.

NB: If you are using a red berry fruit your Kombucha fungus will turn pink! but don't worry about this as they work just as well. We passed one of these funky funguses onto our hairdresser friend whom we knew would appreciate it.

Fruit tea bags can be purchased from a wholefood shop or from a supermarket. Check to make sure that they are real dried fruits and not a concoction of synthetic flavours. Rosehip, hawthorn and blackcurrant are excellent choices and a mixed ginger and apple is also a firm favourite.

FRUITY KOMBUCHA ICED LOLLIES

When one of our local Kombucha network coordinators Kate, in Devon, England, tried fruity Kombucha tea on her children, they seemed to like it. Then one day we were delighted when we were told of the kids latest idea - Kombucha ice-lollies! How wonderful - sucking all that goodness into their bodies.

So, give Kombucha iced lollies a go in the summer months. They can look pretty too, made with raspberry and strawberry flavoured teas. Try them with fresh fruit Kombucha tea (below), and the grown ups will be sucking all that good health in too.

FRESH FRUIT KOMBUCHA TEA

We have had a wonderful time making a variety of beautiful Kombucha drinks in the hot summer days. Here are our two favourites:-

Method

Two days before the end of fermentation purée or liquidise either: 2 fresh mangoes or a punnet of ripe strawberries (or a combination of both). Add to the fermenting Kombucha beverage. The liquid bubbles and froths where a strong fermentation is triggered as soon as the fruit is added. The resulting Kombucha drink is glorious, but we like to improve on this even further: Try adding a splash of elderflower cordial, some sparkling spring water, lots of ice, with maybe a mint leaf or lemon slice. It's heavenly!

When using fresh fruit, the drink will only last 3-4 days in the refrigerator before it starts going off. But this isn't usually a problem, as it disappears long before that anyway! Here is a variety of fruits for you to try: mango, strawberry, raspberry, banana, cooked or raw apple, cherry, blackberry, orange, grape.

KOMBUCHA VINEGAR

If you are brewing your own Kombucha tea for you and your family's health, then it makes sense to make your own high quality vinegar at the same time. It can be used in all kinds of condiments: in salad dressing, mayonnaise, and a variety of sauces. Vinegar tenderises meat and is good on fish and lobster. It helps you to digest tough cellulose, so use it on coarse or stringy cooked vegetables, or sprinkle on raw vegetables.

You can also use Kombucha vinegar to make pickles and preserves and in any recipe that calls for vinegar or cider vinegar. It doesn't have as sharp and acid a flavour as regular processed vinegar does; instead Kombucha vinegar has a richer, rounder and smoother flavour. It is far more pleasant, as well as including Kombucha's beneficial health properties. In fact, Kombucha vinegar's value is much wider, as it can be used in a host of applications:

- for good health
- first-aid
- in the bathroom
- for beauty
- in food recipes
- all around the home
- in the garden

How to Make Kombucha Vinegar

All you do is to allow fermentation to continue up to approximately three weeks, when it will have eventually turned into vinegar. The fermenting time will be more, or less, depending on the warmth of your brewing temperature. Taste it, and if it has a sharp and vinegary tang to it, you're there; if not, leave it for a further 2-3 days and re-taste. Strain and bottle and store away from the light.

Remember to label the Kombucha vinegar so that you won't mix it up with your regular Kombucha tea. It doesn't matter now if you have forgotten a batch of Kombucha tea where it has been left to ferment too long and become sour or vinegary tasting. Just let it go even further and make Kombucha vinegar instead.

Don't be at all put off if you see any kind of streamer-type 'happenings' developing in your vinegar; this only shows that it is a healthy, 'live' and organic substance. All you do is strain these bits off as you pour the vinegar from the bottle when you use it. You may also find a new culture forming on the surface of the bottle. Again this is quite natural and can be left in place, or removed.

Here are some ideas for using Kombucha vinegar:

FRENCH DRESSING

- 1 clove garlic crushed
- 200-ml/⅓-pint (US: 1-cup) of Kombucha vinegar
- 1 tablespoon each honey and dry mustard
- 1 teaspoon each paprika and salt
- 200-ml/ ⅓-pint (US: 1-cup) cold pressed olive oil

Whisk honey, vinegar, mustard, paprika, salt and garlic together until well blended.

Continue whisking and slowly add the olive oil.

KOMBUCHA APPLE DRESSING

This subtle combination of sweet and sour is wonderful with pork, duck, goose or guinea fowl.

- 1 small eating apple, peeled, cored and grated
- 4 tablespoons olive oil
- 2 tablespoons Kombucha vinegar
- 1 teaspoon grain mustard

Put all the ingredients in a screw-top jar and shake well together. Season with salt and pepper to taste.

VINAIGRETTE SAUCE

For cold meats and vegetables;

- 200-ml/⅓-pint (US: 1-cup) each of Kombucha vinegar and cold pressed olive oil
- 1 tablespoon of each:- dry mustard, grated green pepper, chopped parsley, crushed pickles and sugar
- 1 teaspoon each of salt and paprika
- a large pinch of paprika

Mix all the ingredients well and chill. Ideal for summer dishes.

POTATO SALAD

To 450-gms/1-lb (US: 3½-cups) of cooked and diced potatoes add:

- 3 spring onions sliced
- 3 tablespoons fresh parsley
- 2 cloves of garlic chopped fine
- 1 teaspoon of fresh dill chopped fine (or ½-teaspoon dill seed)
- 3 tablespoons finely chopped Kombucha culture

The dressing:

- 5 tablespoons mayonnaise (home made with Kombucha vinegar)
- 1 teaspoon grain mustard
- 2 tablespoons Kombucha vinegar
- salt and pepper to taste

Mix ingredients for the dressing together. Add to the potato, spring onions and garlic while still warm. Toss well. Cover and chill until required. Stir in the parsley, dill and Kombucha culture before serving and adjust seasoning. This will keep for several days in a refrigerator.

Kombucha vinegar used in this recipe, and any other vegetable or pasta salads imparts a lovely flavour, and is much better than using lemon juice or any ordinary vinegar.

FARMER'S PICKLE

(this recipe is adapted and by courtesy of *The Brogdale Apple and Pear Recipe Book.* (See "Recommended Reading")

Ingredients:

- 900-gms/2-lb (US: 7-cups) turnips, peeled and cut into very small cubes
- 450-gms/1-lb (US: 3½-cups) onions, peeled and chopped
- 450-gms/1-lb (US: 3½-cups) apples, peeled, cored and chopped
- 225-gms/8-ozs (US: 1½-cups) raisins
- 225-gms/8-ozs (US: 1½-cups) dark brown sugar
- 14-gms/½ -oz (US: 2 level tablespoons) turmeric

- 50-gms/ 2-ozs (US: 2 rounded tablespoons) sea salt
- 1 teaspoon dry mustard powder
- freshly ground pepper
- 1-litre/2-pints (US: 5-cups) Kombucha vinegar

Method:
Boil turnips in salted water until just cooked, and drain well. Put the cooked turnip, onions, apples, raisins, sugar, salt and pepper into a large pan. Mix turmeric and mustard to a thin paste with some Kombucha vinegar and add to the other ingredients. Bring to the boil and simmer slowly for $1/2$-hour. Stir frequently to avoid sticking. Pour into sterilised jars and cover. Ready to eat 2 two weeks later when it has matured.

KOMBUCHA CHUTNEY
We were given a jar of chutney and recipe by a friend who had made it with ordinary vinegar, but making it ourselves now with Kombucha vinegar has transformed it. All we can say is that it became much smoother, with a gentler taste. Very nice, do try it.

Ingredients:

- 350-gms/12-ozs (US: 2¼-cups) pitted no-soak prunes
- 275-gms/10-ozs (US: 1½-cups) pitted dates
- 275-gms/10-ozs (US: 1½-cups) dried apricots
- 450-gms/1-lb (US: 3½-cups) onions peeled
- 570-mls/1-pint (US: 2½-cups) Kombucha vinegar
- 1 dessertspoon grated fresh root ginger
- 50-gms/2-ozs (US: 2 tablespoons) sea salt
- 75-gms/3-ozs (US: 3 tablespoons) allspice berries
- 450-gms/1-lb (US: 2¼-cups) brown sugar

Method:
Chop dried fruits and onions very small. Tie allspice up in a small piece of muslin and place in a large pan with the vinegar, salt and ginger. Bring to the boil and add the fruits, sugar and onions. Simmer gently for

approximately 1½ hours without a lid or until the chutney has thickened. Stir occasionally to prevent sticking. It is ready when a spoon trail doesn't fill with surplus vinegar. Spoon into sterilised jars, cool and seal. Try and keep this chutney for one month to mature before eating.

ONION VINEGAR
Add 2 small peeled onions to ½-litre/1-pint (US: 2½ -cups) of Kombucha vinegar. Leave covered for three weeks. Remove the onions and use sparingly, a few drops will season most foods.

BEAN SPROUTS
When soaking beansprouts, try soaking them in Kombucha tea instead of water. When sprouted add small pieces of the Kombucha culture cut up to make an unusual and interesting salad.

And what about this wee tip:

ALICK'S KOMBUCHA SOUP STOCK
(Ever The Scotsman!)
When boiling up bones for making stock, add 2 tablespoons of Kombucha vinegar, which will leach out some of the calcium from the bones. In this way you can help prevent osteoporosis and will save money on buying calcium supplement tablets.

FRUIT VINEGARS
USING DRIED FRUITS -
We have made a variety of fruit flavoured vinegars very successfully by making it as in the **Fruit Flavoured Kombucha Tea** method (*See* p.151) - and just allowing it to turn into vinegar. So you can now try raspberry, blackcurrant or rosehip vinegar to make an extra special salad dressing.

USING FRESH FRUITS -
RASPBERRY KOMBUCHA VINEGAR

You will need:

- 250-gms/8-oz (US: 1½-cups) of raspberries
- 570-mls/1-pint (US: 2½ -cups) of Kombucha vinegar

Crush fruit and place in a clean screw top jar with the vinegar. Leave to steep in a warm place for 2-3 weeks shaking the jar occasionally. Strain and pour the fruit vinegar into screw top bottles and label.

ELSIE'S BLACKBERRY VINEGAR
(for those coughs and colds)
This recipe uses fresh fruit to make a healing drink which is excellent if you have a cough or cold, but it can also be drunk as a pleasant hot toddy in the cold days of winter, or to simply enjoy. Can also be drunk as a preventative measure against catching colds!

A kind old lady called Elsie, who came from a Romany family, gave us this recipe, and it has proved to be a firm favourite and a real pleasure to make. Mashing fruits daily, with all the beautiful colours and smells produced, makes this recipe a simple joy. The fruit's beneficial vitamins and flavours will all be preserved and bound together with Kombucha vinegar, making it a most potent combination to heal, soothe and protect.

Method:
Wash the fruit. Blackberry is a favourite, but any other berry such as raspberry or loganberry can be used. Just cover the fruit with Kombucha vinegar in a bowl. Mash the fruit twice a day for 4 days. Strain. Measure the juice and bring it gently to simmering point. For every pint of juice add one pound of sugar (or use honey instead) and stir to dissolve. Bottle and label.

To drink: add 2 tablespoons (or more to taste), of the fruit vinegar to a cup of boiled water and sip slowly.

USING HERBS
HERB VINEGARS
Vinegar has been widely used in the past to enhance the energy and medicinal property of specific plants.

Here are a few suitable herbs that we recommend for you to use; tarragon, savory (winter and summer), basil, marjoram and sage.

You will need:
- a ½-litre/ 1-pint (US: ½-quart) screw-topped jar
- fresh herbs (dried make an inferior taste)
- ½ -litre/1-pint (just under) (US: ½-quart) of Kombucha vinegar

Method:
Pick or buy herbs at their best and bruise with a mortar and pestle (or similar). Add a handful of herbs to the jar and fill to the top with hot (not boiled) Kombucha vinegar. Secure the lid and leave to infuse for 2 weeks. If a stronger flavour is required add another handful of herbs. Leave to infuse for 4 weeks in total. Strain to remove all leaves and stems, and bottle. Screw-tops are preferable to cork, which absorb the flavour of the herb. You can also use a decorative bottle and add a sprig or a few leaves of the herb for decoration. This makes a lovely gift.

Can be used with meat, vegetables, dressings or in cool drinks.

Here a few Kombucha herb vinegars that are useful for first aid and in the home; You may add a few drops - 1 teaspoon of the vinegar to a glass of water:

Peppermint vinegar - calms the digestive system, help cramps, diarrhoea and flatulence. Mixed with honey it is also good for indigestion.

Wormwood vinegar - makes a bitter vinegar, which, when left in a small bowl, will deter flies and other insects. Applied to a wound dressing will assist healing.

Dandelion vinegar - adds a mild laxative element to the vinegar's antiseptic quality. It is rich in potassium, and is known for its help to the pancreas and liver and for lowering blood pressure.

Eucalyptus vinegar - when heated, will release vapours which will help relieve a stuffy head or respiratory tract ("Kombucha inhalation", *see* Chapter 7, "A-Z")

Lavender vinegar - is pleasantly aromatic, and will help nervousness and anxiety.

Myrrh vinegar - swished around the mouth helps to heal sore gums and sweeten the breath. Also for chest congestion.

Rosemary Vinegar - relieves headaches and dizziness, and helps memory.

ROSEMARY AND CRANBERRY DRESSING

This has an exquisite pungent flavour and is delicious with lamb, roasted peppers and aubergines.

Ingredients:

* 1 tablespoon Kombucha vinegar
* 1 sprig of fresh rosemary
* 2 teaspoons cranberry or redcurrant jelly
* 4 tablespoons olive oil

Method:

In a thick saucepan heat the vinegar, jelly and rosemary slowly until the jelly has dissolved. Remove from heat and cool. Gradually whisk in the olive oil and season with salt and pepper. This dressing can be served warm.

BEAUTY

THE SKIN

Kombucha tea grows a new layer of skin (culture) each time that we feed it with a nutrient solution, and in return proves itself to be effective as a wonderful health and healing product for *all* skin conditions. It is extremely beneficial in medical conditions such as eczema, acne, psoriasis and leg ulcers. It is equally good in the natural cosmetics field.

The skin reflects how and who we are, through our ups and downs, emotions and health in life. Skin is more than just a cover, it is the body's largest organ; it regulates body temperature, provides a protective barrier against bacteria and eliminates toxins from the body. If our skin allows toxins out, then it can certainly allow other substances in. A clove of garlic rubbed onto the sole of the foot of a baby could be smelt on its breath ten minutes later. This shows that the substance had passed through the skin, entered the bloodstream and returned via the lungs and onto the breath.

This example shows how important it is to be aware of the substances that we place in contact with our skin. Everything that is able to permeate the skin layer will enter the body system from atmosphere, baths, washing, creams, massage etc. We can therefore assume that the natural Kombucha beauty therapy will be working its benefits towards our inner body, as well as helping our outer skin.

The skin has a certain amount of natural acidity. A healthy skin will produce its own acid mantle again after a few hours of washing with soap which has rendered it alkaline. Constant washing, pollution, the sun and centrally heated environments make our skin dull, dry, lifeless and unable to function properly. Kombucha is such a beneficial skin aid because it matches the skin's acidity, and helps to keep it looking fresh, youthful and glowing.

Kombucha is unsurpassed and has been used for centuries. So rediscover nature's way and save a fortune on the many expensive beauty aids that it will replace. Here are some very effective ways that we can use Kombucha for the skin:-

KOMBUCHA TEA BATH

What better way to relax than in a warm Kombucha bath when we want to let go of the day and be uplifted. Add 1-2 litres/2-4 pints (US: 5-10 cups) of Kombucha tea to the bath just before entering. You will feel a tingle on the skin and if there is a little smarting in the eyes, it will quickly pass, leaving them cleansed and refreshed too. There is no need to use soap, instead use a good brush or loofah to loosen dirt, clear away old dead skin scales and leave your skin feeling soft, fresh and revitalised.

KOMBUCHA MASSAGE

One of Kombucha tea's many fascinating properties is that it relieves tiredness and can be used as a full or partial massage. Try this next time you feel exhausted after a workday hunched over a desk:

Add 2 cups of Kombucha tea or 1 cup of Kombucha vinegar into a small bowl of warm water and massage it several times vigorously over the back, neck, shoulders and arms or give yourself the full body treatment in a bath tub or shower. Allow the liquid to dry naturally on the skin without washing it off. This will pep you up and give you new vitality, which is welcome after a tiring day and before an enjoyable evening out.

KOMBUCHA SPONGE

While you are in the bath or shower, you could use one of your spare funguses as a sponge to give yourself a Kombucha rub-down. It will leave your body toned, invigo-rated and tingling all over; just the thing on a dull day. Small funguses or pieces can also be used on the face using small circular movements and long strokes on the neck. If you have a sensitive skin, rinse the fungus under the tap or in a bowl of water to dilute it slightly, as it contains Kombucha in a quite concentrated form.

KOMBUCHA TEA CLEANSER/ASTRINGENT/TONER

Kombucha tea is a wonderful all-in-one cleanser, astringent and toner for the skin, leaving it feeling fresh, smooth and soft. Use in proportion of 1:3, ie ¼ volume of water, to ¾ volume of Kombucha tea, which brings the acid balance close to the skin's natural pH, otherwise it may be too strong for some skin types. So, throw away all those different bottles and have just one costing next to nothing. The slight tangy smell soon evaporates used on its own or create an aromatic by adding flowers:

FRESH FLOWER KOMBUCHA TEA CLEANSER/ASTRINGENT/TONER

* 3 tablespoons lavender flowers*
* 425-mls/³/₄ -pint (US: a little over 2¼ - cups) Kombucha tea
* 150-mls/¼-pint (US: ¾-cup) of water - preferably rainwater, or try rose or or-ange water**

Add flowers to Kombucha tea and steep for 2 weeks, strain and add water. Pour into decorative bottle.
* rose petals, violets, rose geranium, lemon verbena, bergamot, rosemary and camomile can be used; also elderflower which lightens skin and fades freckles.
** available from most chemists and drug stores

KOMBUCHA TEA STEAM FACIAL

Steaming will loosen dirt and grease and deep-clean the pores. It can be used daily for normal to oily skins and fortnightly for dry skin types.

* 200-mls/¹/₃-pint (US: 1-cup) of Kombucha tea
* 1-litre/2-pints (US: 5-cups) of boiling wa-ter in a bowl.

Pour boiling water into a bowl and add the Kombucha tea. Put your face over the bowl and cover your head and the bowl with a towel to create a hood. Allow the steam to soak your face for 10 minutes or more. Now apply Kombucha tea Toner and rest. Don't go outside for at least 2 hours until your open pores and bronchial tubes have re-turned to normal again.

NB: People with broken facial veins should avoid this method.

KOMBUCHA FACE MASK

There is a wide range of natural plant sub-stances that can be used to maximum bene-fit in their fresh state to cleanse and enhance the condition of our facial skin.

Here are some ideas:

* A Kombucha culture put through a blender and applied to the face makes an invigorating face mask, or add it to a beaten white of egg for oily skin or yolk of egg for dry skin.

* Mix some Kombucha tea with uncooked (not runny) honey, to make a remarkable healing medium that will moisturise, stimulate and soothe the skin.

* Blend or mash a Papaya (Paw Paw) fruit which contains an enzyme that can sof-ten protein tissue. Mix with Kombucha tea and apply to the face. Wash off after 5 minutes only, as it is quite strong and dry the face with a soft cloth.

First cleanse the skin using a Kombucha tea steam facial or Kombucha tea cleanser. Gen-tly pat the ingredients on to your face. Al-low 20-30 minutes for them to do their work while lying down quietly with your feet raised up. Wash off the mask with cotton wool or a soft flannel and tepid water. Close the pores with Kombucha tea astringent.

If a mixture is too runny, or as an alternative facial mask, add any of the following binding substances; banana, avocado, fresh strawberries, honey, fullers earth, oatmeal, whole egg, egg white, egg yolk for dry skin, yoghurt.

Some facial masks can also be effective on other parts of the body, such as elbows, knees, feet, legs and buttocks which may have dried skin. So use any leftovers and restore these parts of the body too. Ingredients can be stored in the refrigerator for several days.

KOMBUCHA CREAM

Creams offer a versatile medium to apply Kombucha to any part of the skin where its healing properties are needed. Cut the fungus into small pieces and pulverise in an electric blender until it is fine and pulped. Add it to any base skin cream that you may have, which provides a barrier for the skin, and a medium to allow Kombucha's healing properties to work. (*See* "Resources and Suppliers")

KOMBUCHA DEODORANT

Many people who are allergic to commercial deodorants can try splashing on the *Kombucha Tea Cleanser/Astringent/Toner* which has anti-bacterial properties. It is very effective in restoring the skin's natural pH and, though you still perspire naturally, there is less odour.

KOMBUCHA AFTERSHAVE

This is a good bactericide aftershave and will prevent 'barber's rash'.

- 250-mls/ 9-fl.oz. (US: 1¼-cups) orange-flower water
- 25-mls/1-fl.oz. (US: 2-tablespoons) vodka
- 10-mls/1-dessertspoon (US: 2-teaspoons) Kombucha vinegar
- 6 drops Sandalwood or other suitable essential oil

Combine all ingredients and bottle.

WRINKLES AND CROWS' FEET

Kombucha has been reported historically as removing wrinkles, improving skin condition and helping one to look younger. This has been borne out by many women who swear to its efficacy in association with taking it internally. Try it yourself:

Apply Kombucha tea Toner or Cream around the eyes, neck and chest twice daily to soften and smooth the skin.

SCARS

Kombucha tea or Cream applied regularly will heal the skin and gradually fade a minor scar.

BROWN LIVER SPOTS

Kombucha tea helps the removal of brown (liver) spots on the hands; apply it with a pad of cotton wool morning and evening. Try the Kombucha Tea Toner made with elderflower which will give the added benefits of being good for fading freckles and lightening the skin.

KOMBUCHA MOUTHWASH

Kombucha tea on its own is a refreshing and effective mouthwash. Here is another recipe that will make the mouth come alive:

- 250-mls/9-fl.oz (US: 1¼-cups) of Kombucha tea
- add to it essential oils; 30 drops each Thyme and Peppermint and 10 drops each of Fennel and Myrrh.

Put all the ingredients into a bottle and shake well. Add 2-3 teaspns to half a glass of warm water and rinse the mouth as required.

HAIR

The health of the hair and scalp depends to a great extent on our general health and nutrition. A balanced diet providing essential vitamins and minerals goes a long way in keeping our hair looking strong and shiny. Kombucha tea provides much of this nutrition and in addition both the tea and vinegar have proved to be a wonderful hair tonic. With its high acidity Kombucha contains powerful enzymes which kill the bottle bacillus, a germ responsible for starving hair follicles of oil and causing many scalp and skin conditions including itching, dandruff and thinning hair.

Drinking Kombucha tea has returned grey hair to its former colour with some people, but not all. You could always give it a try and see what happens!

KOMBUCHA HAIR RINSE

Commercial shampoos are usually alkaline; the scalp on the other hand is acid and is protected by natural oils. This, however, is washed away, allowing the skin to become scaly and the scalp dry. The balance can be restored by using Kombucha after you have shampooed your hair. This method has proved very effective for all kinds of dry hair, scalp and skin conditions:

As a final hair rinse pour 1-cup of Kombucha tea over hair and leave for at least 15 minutes and up to 2-3 hours in chronic conditions. Cover head with a plastic bag and towel. Rinse and repeat weekly or more if necessary.

Try a maceration of rosemary and nettles for greasy hair (also good for darkening) in the rinsing water or add a few drops of essential oil of rosemary.

KOMBUCHA HAIR CONDITIONER

This is a fresh-smelling and effective conditioner:

* 25-gms/ 1-oz (1 rounded tablespoon) fresh rosemary or 12-grams/ ½-oz dried (US: ¼-cup fresh or 1-teaspoon dried)
* 275-mls/½-pint (US: 1¼-cups) water (rain is best)
* 275-mls/½-pint (US: 1¼-cups) of Kombucha vinegar

Bring water slowly to the boil and add rosemary. Simmer for 10 minutes, strain and mix with Kombucha vinegar. When cooled, pour into bottles and store in a cool dark place. After washing hair, dry and pour a little into the palm of the hands and rub vigorously into hair and scalp with the finger tips.

KOMBUCHA SHAMPOO

Make your own shampoo by adding some Kombucha vinegar to your own favourite

shampoo in a ratio of 1:10. Use as normal shampoo. In this way you can have your shampoo and conditioner all in one bottle. With regular use you will develop a good body, condition and shine to your hair. Hairdressers the world over recognise the importance of using a shampoo with natural plant substances that will not strip your hair of natural oils, and will match the skin's natural pH on your head. Some hairdressers have discovered Kombucha shampoo. It is effective and it costs a lot less too!

DANDRUFF

Apply Kombucha tea or vinegar soaked in a pad of cotton wool directly to the scalp by parting the hair in sections. Leave for at least 15 minutes and up to 3 hours before shampooing for acute cases. This should be done before each shampoo.

HAIR LOSS (*See* Chapter 7, "A-Z")

EYES

Our eyes are a reflection of our body health, especially the liver and gall bladder and will a have a yellow look if those organs are not working well. Black rings and puffiness under the eyes indicates that our kidneys are out of balance and that we are tired. Our eyes show the world our joy or sadness and are a mirror to the soul.

While Kombucha can be effective to a certain extent as an external aid, it is obvious that a healthily functioning body will produce healthy eyes. This is why we welcome Kombucha tea in association with a balanced diet and good exercise.

KOMBUCHA EYEBATH

Add 1 teaspoon of eyebright herb to a cup of boiled water and allow to steep for 10 minutes. Strain and cool the liquid in the refrigerator. Add 1 teaspoon of Kombucha vinegar or 2 teaspoons of Kombucha tea, soak 2 small pads of cottonwool and place over the eyes; rest for at least 1 hour, lying down. If you do not have any eyebright this may be omitted and Kombucha used on its own to excellent effect.

PUFFY EYES

Use Kombucha tea Toner using a pad of cotton wool around the eyes, or Kombucha cream, but avoid the eyes themselves.

WEIGHT LOSS (*See* Chapter 7, "A-Z")

SPRING TONIC

After the long, dark, days of winter when we have been sitting around, eating more and exercising less, we will benefit enormously from a spring-time cleanse. When the new shoots of the herbs dandelion and stinging nettle begin peeping through the ground, then is the time. These bitter herbs are our spring-cleaners and blood purifiers and, in addition to Kombucha, make a potent drink that will put the spring back into your step.

KOMBUCHA TEA SPRING CLEANSE

When making Kombucha tea, substitute half the green or black tea with a mixture of fresh young dandelion leaves and nettle tops (careful, wear gloves). As a guideline use twice as much fresh herbs as you would dried or tea.

You can drink the Kombucha tea Spring Cleanse as usual instead of Kombucha tea, or you might like to go on a mild fast. This will help to give the body an extra clean-out and also tackle the extra weight that has accumulated over the winter months.

- Substitute one meal a day - lunch or evening, with a glass of Kombucha tea Spring Cleanse for 2-3 weeks.
- *Or* drink Kombucha tea Spring Cleanse one day a week (Monday is good) to replace meals for the whole day; again do this for 2-3 weeks.

BODY BUILDING

In Harald Tietze's book *Kombucha - Miracle Fungus*, he describes how the Russian military regularly drink Kombucha, and in Germany, particular regiments have their secret Kombucha recipes. Russian high performance athletes were given Kombucha tea, and in scientific tests after hard training, showed the following results:

- performances were notably improved
- muscular aches and pains were reduced
- athletes recovered quicker after exertion
- salt in lactic acid was noticeably reduced

The conclusion they came to was that, "This pure biological Kombucha fermented tea had a strengthening effect and improved the performances of the athletes".

Athletes in general would notice an increase in energy and a refreshing drink along at the gym could be $\frac{1}{2}$ Kombucha tea and $\frac{1}{2}$ carbonated water, which can replace an expensive commercial sports drink. If quick weight loss is the goal then substituting a glass of Kombucha tea for lunch can be very effective.

KOMBUCHA IN THE HOME

Kombucha has a role in all areas of our lives where it cleans and heals the body and no less can also clean and heal our homes. The valuable use of Kombucha in its vinegar form for cleaning in the home has been chronicled for hundreds of years. Here are but a few recommendations (*See* p.152 above, on "How to make Kombucha Vinegar") NB: Remember to use green tea.

KOMBUCHA AIR FRESHENER

Mix together 1 tablespoon of Kombucha vinegar with 1 teaspoon of baking soda in 400-mls/$\frac{2}{3}$-pint (US: 2-cups) of water. When the foaming stops, screw on the top and shake well. For instant freshness, spray into the room. Add a few drops of Bergamot oil for a delicious, uplifting, citrusy fragrance which can appeal to both sexes.

COOKING ODOURS

To clear the air of lingering cooking odours, simmer 200-mls/$\frac{1}{3}$-pint (US: 1-cup) of Kombucha vinegar in an uncovered pot of water to which 1 teaspoon cinnamon has been added. Simmer slowly for approx. $\frac{1}{2}$ hour, or longer if necessary.

CLEARS UP PAINT SMELLS

Leave a dish or two of Kombucha vinegar around when painting and decorating to absorb the odours.

KOMBUCHA WINDOW CLEANER
Mix 2-tablespoons of Kombucha vinegar with 570-mls/1-pint (US: 2½-cups) water in a pump spray bottle. This makes an effective window cleaner; just spray onto the glass and wipe off immediately with a clean, soft cloth.

KOMBUCHA FURNITURE POLISH
For a light polish use 1 part lemon oil to 3 parts Kombucha vinegar. For a heavy polish use 3 parts oil and 1 part vinegar. The vinegar dissolves the dirt and the oil nourishes the wood. For dusting, dampen cloth with half Kombucha vinegar and half olive oil. The wood will come up clean and sweet smelling.

CLEAN AND PRESERVE LEATHER SHOES
Mix 1-tablespoon of alcohol, 1-tablespoon of Kombucha vinegar, 1-teaspoon liquid soap and 1 teaspoon vegetable oil. Wipe on to clean and then brush or buff to shine.

KOMBUCHA BRASS AND COPPER POLISH
To 2-teaspoons of salt mix 1-tablespoon of flour. Add enough Kombucha vinegar to make a thick paste. Add more salt for tough jobs or more flour and vinegar for a softer paste. Scrub the metal with a small brush, rinse and buff to shine.

KOMBUCHA DISINFECTANT
Wipe all kitchen and bathroom surfaces with Kombucha vinegar to clean, disinfect and prevent mould.

KOMBUCHA TOILET CLEANER
Pour Kombucha vinegar over stained area in the bowl and sprinkle borax over the vinegar. Leave for 2 hours, then brush and flush.

KOMBUCHA LIMESCALE REMOVER
Mix 1 teaspoon of alum (aluminium sulphate) in 55-mls/ 2-fl.ozs (US: ¼-cup) of Kombucha vinegar. Wipe on the bath or shower door and scrub with a soft brush. Rinse with lots of water and polish until

dry. We have cleaned our shower head and kettle very effectively by soaking for 2 hours in Kombucha vinegar only. Loosen limescale with a small brush and rinse clean.

CLEANING AND FRESHENING
Add 4 tablespoons of Kombucha vinegar to hot water for cleaning work surfaces and floors; it will add sparkle and freshness. Adding to a load of laundry with the usual soap will brighten colours and make whites shine.

REMOVES SCUM
Add a cup of Kombucha vinegar to a bucket of clear water after washing the floor, to rinse and prevent a dull scum. Makes floors clean and shining bright

CLEANS WOODEN CUTTING BOARDS
Wipe down wooden boards with full strength Kombucha vinegar to clean, cut grease and absorb odours.

WASHING-UP
1-cup of Kombucha vinegar added to dish washing water cuts through grease and lets you use less soap. Also soak or simmer stuck or burnt on food by adding 2-cups of water and 1-cup of vinegar. The food will soften and lift off in 5-10 minutes.

CLEANS BABIES' TOYS
Add a generous splash of Kombucha vinegar to soapy water when cleaning and disinfecting babies' toys. Rinse well.

CLEANING VEGETABLES
Add a little vinegar and salt to the vegetable rinsing water to lift out bugs and kill germs.

FOR HARDENED PAINT BRUSHES
Put 150-mls/ ¼-pint (US: ¾-cup) Kombucha vinegar in a large food can and add brushes. Simmer over a low heat for 20-mins. Rinse well, working the softened paints out of the brushes. In worst cases a second treatment may be necessary.

HAIRBRUSHES
Clean brushes by adding 1-cup of Kombucha vinegar in 2-cups of hot soapy water.

CHAPTER 14

ANIMALS AND PLANTS

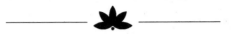

While Kombucha can prove very beneficial to an animal's health, it does not take the place of medical supervision by your veterinary surgeon.

There have been many remarkable stories of how animals have benefited from the wonderful healing properties of Kombucha. There is every reason to include Kombucha therapy in a programme of health care for our fellow creatures who deserve as much love and attention to their well-being as we humans do. This can easily be done by adding Kombucha tea, vinegar or the actual fungus to an animal's daily diet.

In the case of an actual illness, Kombucha can be applied in a whole variety of ways as we have described in the "A-Z" and "First Aid" chapters.

Relief can be gained from many chronic and acute health problems, including skin complaints, allergies, arthritis, liver, the stomach, kidneys etc. If we remember that our pets can suffer from similar causes for their illnesses as we do, this can give us insights on how to help them.

Here are some possible causes for an animal's illness:
- it doesn't have a good diet - eats processed foods, mostly out of tins. Not the kind of food that it would be able to obtain in the wild.
- it is unable to have the right healing herbs and plants that it would instinctively eat in the wild, to help a malady.
- it is over-fed and over-weight
- it doesn't get enough exercise
- it suffers degeneration due to poor living accommodation
- it leads a boring and unfulfilled life
- it suffers from an emotional problem due to living circumstances or abuse
- its health is declining due to the ageing process
- it isn't loved and listened to enough (all animals communicate)

Accidents and Injuries
Cats and dogs often get injured in fights over territory, or by a car when crossing the road. An accident can happen in a field in the quiet countryside, as the following story tells:

This much loved young animal almost didn't see beyond its first six months of life. It is a story which needs spreading about far and wide, showing us all, including veterinary surgeons, that there are other ways instead of, and if antibiotics fail.

SUNRAY'S STORY
Shirley Bitton (*See* Case Study, p.124), who ran an animal shelter on holistic

lines for 15 years, clearly has a natural affinity for animals. This showed itself in 1995 when a 4-month old pure Arab foal called Sunray, got a very deep cut in its hind leg. The vet treated this with several different courses of antibiotics without any sign of improvement, and the foal's health steadily deteriorated. After three months of this treatment, and with the ugly wound still suppurating and becoming worse than ever, the vet eventually recommended that nothing else could be done and the foal be put down. Shirley herself did not believe that the foal would survive until the next day because it was so ill. But, being a healer, she was searching for anything that might help, before giving up on the life of this vulnerable creature.

The next morning an idea came to her. She had read that the Kombucha fungus has been used with success topically on hard to heal leg ulcers, and maybe it would help Sunray. Three people eventually managed to place a fungus on the foal's leg and strap it up with a bandage. It was obvious from its writhing that the smarting was giving him a lot of pain, but it was a case of 'kill-or-cure' at this stage, and the stinging gradually eased.

The next day when they removed the dressing, they found that an enormous amount of puss had drained out, and the fungus had dried and shrivelled to a thin film. Much of the moisture, and healing properties from the big fungus they had applied would have entered into the wound.

They then applied a new Kombucha fungus and a fresh dressing to the leg. The following day the pus had stopped suppurating and a healing skin had started to form around the outside of the lesion. After one week of daily changing the Kombucha poultice, the wound completely healed, and the horse was literally prancing around with new energy. Kombucha tea had also been added to his food, and this was continued after the leg had healed. There is no sign of injury at all now on Sunray's leg, and he lives a healthy and happy life with four strong and sturdy legs.

It is very sad indeed when our beloved animal whom we have lived with, and has become a companion and confidante, eventually becomes seriously ill. We want to do all we possibly can to save its life or make its remaining days as comfortable and as happy as possible. This is the least we can do, after a lifetime of their devoted and unconditional service to us.

PRINCE'S TALE

In 1997 the Bitton's golden retriever Prince who, at 11 years old, was suffering from bone cancer, got secondary skin cancer in his foreleg. This was removed by surgery, but left a sore that wouldn't heal with antibiotics and was still suppurating after one month.

Shirley made up her mind that she would try Kombucha on Prince too, to see if this would help him as much as it had done with Sunray. The position of the wound made it hard to apply a dressing, so she lay down with the dog in the evening, holding a Kombucha fungus over the sore. Within 3 days it was healed, and on the fourth day, the stitches were able to be taken out.

Prince has now become partial to Kombucha and loves to eat bits of the culture, which Shirley hopes might also help with his bone cancer. We hope so too.

Shirley says that; "Friends who heard about our experiences have brought sheep with footrot, which we have treated successfully with a Kombucha poultice, as well as other horses with more minor cuts and grazes than Sunray's, but all with very good results".

Placebos Don't Work with Animals

In trials conducted on humans, it has generally been found that as a rule of thumb, up to $\frac{1}{3}$rd of people who have been given an inert alternative to the remedy they thought that they had been given, showed some improvement in their health. However as animals don't imagine as we do or are governed by their psychological processes, placebos will not work on them. So when Kombucha therapy or a homoeopathic remedy works on an animal, as they often do, this proves their efficacy quite objectively.

Animals also benefit from a Holistic Approach

Whilst Kombucha can help the symptomatic relief of an animal's health problems, the underlying cause needs addressing also.

Kombucha can be given internally to animals to strengthen their body functioning and overall health in the usual ways, but with some adjustments if they find it unpalatable. Amounts need to be adjusted according to animal type and size.

Here are a few ways of giving Kombucha:
• Kombucha tea can be added to drinking water. Experiment and find the amount that your animal will tolerate. If, for example, a cat or dog won't take it in water, adding it to milk will often be acceptable. Add only a few drops of Kombucha tea to the drinking water of a very small animal, such as a hamster, but up to ½ -1 gallon (US: 5-10-pints) may be added to the drinking water of a horse or cow, and half this amount for a goat.
• A Kombucha culture may be chopped up in an animal's food, or just given in small pieces in its natural state from the hand like a tit-bit (many dogs will take it like this).
• Kombucha tea may be added to the feed of pigs, sheep and cattle. With horses and ponies, it may be advisable to give it with their favourite food, as they can be slightly fussy eaters.

ANIMAL HEALTH - RECOMMENDATIONS AND ADVICE

These recommendations are from some Kombucha brewers on The Kombucha Tea Network UK who have found while improving their own and their family's health, they wanted to extend this further to the wider family of their animal friends.

You may find that what works for one animal, though individual, may be applied to another:

FLEAS

During the flea season spray either full strength Kombucha tea or diluted with water 3:1 (3 parts Kombucha tea/1 part water), on irritated and sore areas of an animal's skin where they have been scratching badly. Protect the animal's eyes when spraying.

NB: While this remedy helps to heal and soothe the irritation, we are unable to say at present if this will actually kill or deter the fleas themselves, which are the cause of the problem, and obviously need treating.

BALD PATCHES
Apply Kombucha tea onto the skin at least twice a day with a pad of cotton wool and allow to dry.

SWOLLEN AND BLEEDING GUMS
This method was applied to a cat whose gums were badly infected, and they apparently cleared up in three days. Using a small syringe (available from chemists and drug stores), squirt Kombucha tea into the sides of the mouth, 2 - 3 times a day.

DIARRHOEA
Kombucha tea was given to a small dog by syringe and relief was experienced very quickly, after having had several days of 'the runs' (diarrhoea).

SORES AND CUTS
Bathe, to clean the wound with Kombucha tea, using a pad of cottonwool. Apply fresh Kombucha tea to the affected area 2 - 3 times per day. Allow it to dry naturally, or apply a Kombucha compress or poultice, and secure with a dressing and change daily.

AGEING ANIMALS
Several people have reported to us how their elderly dogs and cats have shown a significant improvement in health and vitality after being given Kombucha. Skin has improved and coats become glossy, in addition to brighter eyes. Other senses had improved with an overall increase in energy.

TUMOURS
We were told of a cat 15 years old who had a tumour, and was given 1 teaspoon of Kombucha tea in its water every day. Its energy improved to the point of being quite kittenish, and its bowel movements returned to normal.

NEW LIFE!
It is well worth trying Kombucha with an animal who has been given up on by the vet. This account came from a delighted pet owner whose 10 year old Pekinese dog was very ill, and considered to be dying. Euthanasia had been suggested by the vet and declined by the owner. Animals, like children, can respond very quickly. We were told that this particular dog made a remarkable turnaround in health, and to the amazement of all, was running around very soon after being given Kombucha tea for a couple of weeks.

HORSES' AND PONIES' COATS
Their condition can be improved we are told, through a course of Kombucha, bringing a bloom and suppleness.

INFLUENZA AND COUGHS
It has been suggested quite rightly that a regular intake of Kombucha tea can build up a healthy immunity for many animals who may suffer from these types of illnesses; notably horses, cats and dogs.

RESTORING HEALTHY INTESTINAL FUNCTIONING
This aspect is especially important when an animal has been on a course of antibiotics, which damage healthy bacteria in the gut. Kombucha can help restore normal health and functioning to the digestion and intestinal processes.

DUNG EATING
This unpleasant habit can be caused by a nutritional deficiency, and may be corrected through proper diet, including Kombucha, which contains beneficial minerals and vitamins which are often lacking in an animals food.

KOMBUCHA AND THE FARMER
We have a lot of interest and enquiries about Kombucha from farm workers. Kombucha can prove very effective for the health of animals on the farm, both in preventative care and in treatment. Here are some recommendations:

POULTRY
The shell texture of eggs may be improved with the addition of Kombucha vinegar to their feed or drinking water.

ARTHRITIS AND RHEUMATISM
Cows who have become lame and stiff can be given a longer active and milk producing life when on a regular Kombucha regime.

DYSENTERY
A cow can be given 110mls/4-fl.ozs (US: ½-cup) of Kombucha vinegar in 275mls /½-pint (US: 1¼-cups) of warm water twice a day by the bottle until an improvement is seen, and the animal is successfully chewing the cud again. Kombucha tea or vinegar can then be added to the drinking water.

DIGESTION
Many animals, including cattle, sheep and deer have very complex digestive systems to process the large amounts of cellulose they eat, which contain specialised bacteria in the alimentary canal. Antibiotics can upset the balance and lead to a loss of appetite and a halt in cudding. The organic acids, including acetic acid in Kombucha, replace and assist normal bacterial action, proper functioning of the rumen, and ensure a healthy digestive system.

For poor appetite, give by bottle feed until appetite is restored;
• adult animal 100-mls/4-fl.ozs (US: ½-cup) Kombucha vinegar twice per day in 300-mls/½-pint (US: 2½-cups) warm water
• younger animals (bulling age) 50-mls/2-fl.ozs (US: 4-tablespoons) once a day in 300mls/½-pint (US: 2½-cups) warm water

- weaned calves 25-mls/1-fl.oz (US: 2-tablespoons) once a day in 150-mls/¼-pint (US: 1¼-cups) warm water
- new born calves 2 teaspoons a day in 150-mls/¼-pint (US: 1¼cups) warm water

ACID-ALKALI BALANCE

The correct balance in an animal's body chemistry is of vital importance, as all farmers know, in building up resistance to many illnesses on the farm. The acid/alkaline balance can be improved through regular intake of Kombucha.

KOMBUCHA IN THE GARDEN

Kombucha is becoming more widely used and its success has now spread 'organically' into the garden! Based on the understanding that Kombucha's antiseptic properties kill harmful bacteria in the human body, it will have a similar effect with your garden plants and pests. This will be in a way that is natural, will do no harm to the environment or ecosystem, and will actually improve the health of the plant and soil along the way.

The following recommendations have been passed on to you by two co-ordinators from the Kombucha Tea Network UK who have found them to be very successful.

KOMBUCHA FUNGICIDE

(this comes from Bob Banham in East Anglia, UK)

Mildew, which is a greyish, powdery-looking coating, is usually seen on young stalks and leaves of plants. Spray full strength Kombucha tea at the first sign. Respray if necessary.

This was done to courgette plants that were in quite a bad state in the greenhouse, and within a couple of days they had picked up dramatically and went on to grow and produce well. Bob, who is an experienced gardener, said that previously, if mildew had occurred to the extent that his plants were affected, they would normally have died.

NB: It is important to treat mildew quickly, as it can spread rapidly.

KOMBUCHA AND GARLIC INSECT SPRAY

(and this recipe comes from Barbara Bruce in the Channel Islands)

For insects, caterpillars etc. make a Kombucha garlic water spray; by crushing 1 clove of garlic in 1-litre/2-pints (US: 2½-pints) of hot water and then bottle. Leave for 4 days and strain (so garlic doesn't block spray), add 1 squirt of washing-up liquid and 150-mls/¼-pint (US: ¾-cup) of Kombucha tea. Spray vegetables. Once or twice is usually enough, but re-apply if there is any further infestation. Barbara also recommends that burying a retired Kombucha fungus near an old fruit tree will be beneficial to it!

SOIL

Adding old Kombucha funguses, which contain concentrated Kombucha, to an alkaline soil will change the pH to a more acid state (but don't do this if your soil is already acidic!). This will be of benefit to acid loving plants such as azaleas, rhododendrons, pieris, skimmias etc.

TREES

In 1961 Dr med. Valentin Koehler's research took him from the realms of treating cancer patients with Kombucha containing glucuronic acid which has a detoxification role in the human body, to that of nature and trees. He stated that, "Here is a possible aid for a humanity that is more and more threatened through toxic environmental substances, and .... by glucuronic acid the disturbance products in the human body are disintegrated into end-products, eliminated and made harmless, and lastly .... glucuronic acid bene-fits cellular functions."

With regards trees he described glucuronic acid as having the capacity to enter into combination with both foreign and endogenic toxic substances and to protect the plant cell. He said that over 200 substances can be made harmless this way, including those which are contained in acidic and radio-active rain, as well as sulphur dioxide and nitrite. Dr Koehler explains that the protective activity connected with glucuronic acid will also preserve the genetics of a plant from growth disturbances and will promote their restora-tion in the further course of its growth.

So what does this mean?

We would recommend watering trees and shrubs in a proportion of $\frac{1}{2}$ -litre/1-pint (US: $\frac{1}{2}$-quart) of Kombucha tea to 4-litres/1-gall. (US: 10-pints) of water (preferably rainwater from a water butt). Mulch around the base to conserve the moisture. Repeat every 2 - 3 weeks throughout the growing season. Kombucha tea spray can be applied directly onto the leaves, in a proportion of 1:3, Kombucha tea and water.

We are getting reports from Kombucha brewers who have discovered (often accidentally) that a Kombucha culture buried near the roots can have beneficial results for an ailing plant. In one case an unhealthy bush put out new growth within 3 weeks, and in another a holly tree suffering from scale seemed to throw it off in a similar time.

PLANT POTS

Clean and disinfect your plant pots naturally by washing them in 4-pints of hot water to which 1-cup of Kombucha vinegar has been added.

There is a lot of food for thought here, so garden lovers - please do ex-periment using Kombucha tea in watering and sprays, with compost heaps and sick plants, shrubs and trees etc. Do let's have some feedback so that we can spread the word in future editions, and all of us expand our knowledge of using Kombucha in the animal and plant kingdoms.

PLEASE GIVE US YOUR FEEDBACK ON KOMBUCHA

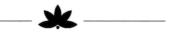

We believe that Kombucha therapy has an important part to play in the healing of our society. In the free giving of spare Kombucha cultures to our family, friends and neighbours, we are also helping to build caring communities.

We would like to see a wider sharing and awareness of reliable Kombucha information, so we propose to start a Kombucha newsletter. We would like to publish letters and articles of interest from Kombucha users which we feel would inspire and benefit others. If you would be interested in receiving the newsletter, please contact us for further information, by sending an s.a.e..

If you have found this book useful, please send us your own experience and insights and relevant feedback. We would also be very interested to hear from doctors and practitioners who have used Kombucha therapy with their patients.

The Kombucha Network UK has a page on the Gateway Books Website: **www// gatewaybooks.com**

Please write to us at: **The Kombucha Tea Network UK**, PO Box 1887, Bath, BA2 8YA.   Thank you, and Good Health!

Alick and Mari Bartholomew

GLOSSARY

Acetic acid The scientific name for vinegar.

Acid 1 -6·5 is acid on pH scale. More acid means greater number of hydrogen ions present.

Acidosis Excessive acidity of body fluids; worst foods - beer, wine, coffee, fatty foods.

Acute illness Sudden and of limited duration.

Adaptogen A substance which returns the body metabolism (qv) to balance.

Alkaline 7·1 -14 on the pH scale; foods which encourage alkalinity - complex carbohydrates and proteins.

Amino acids Protein-based substances which work closely with enzymes. In Kombucha the sulphur-based ones are vital in their ability to rid body of toxic chemicals and heavy metals through the liver.

Antibiotic The principal method of fighting infections, originally using chemically synthesised varieties of penicillin (discov.1940), derived from bacteria and moulds; term also used for drugs to counter protozoal and fungal infections.

Bacteria Simplest form of cell organisms.

Bacterioides The less acid intestinal bacteria responsible for putrefaction of food; encouraged by diet high in fats & proteins; need to be balanced by bifidobacteria.

Balancer (see Adaptogen)

Bifidobacteria Beneficial producers of acetic, lactic and folic acids encouraged by diet strong in carbohydrate, fibre and lacto-vegetarian food.

Butyric acid Protects cellular membranes. Working symbiotically (qv) with caprylic acid (see Gluconic) counters candidiasis. Also a disinfectant.

Candida albicans (candidiasis) A yeast which in its pathological form depletes the immune function and contributes to chronic illnesses.

Chronic illness = long lasting.

Chronic Fatigue Syndrome (Myalgic Encephalomyelitis or ME) A chronic condition with muscular pain and stiffness, swollen glands, headaches and profound pain - of viral origin, sometimes persisting for up to 30 years.

Collagen A fibrous protein responsible for connective tissue.

Detoxifier Any substance which captures toxins in the liver to release them to the kidneys for elimination.

DNA The carrier of genetic information to all organisms.

Dysbiosis A state of disorganisation which allows illness to develop.

Endocrine glands are part of the immune system.

Energy medicine Medical treatments which work at a non-physical, energy level eg acupuncture, homoeopathy, shiatsu.

Epidermal cells are hardened by the protein keratin as they migrate to the skin surface. If this happens too fast a skin disorder occurs called psoriasis.

Essiac (The Rene Caisse Herbal Mixture) The Canadian Ojibway Indians' remedy for cancer prevention and treatment, combining the herbs sheep sorrel, burdock root, slippery elm and Turkish rhubarb root.

Ethanol a grain alcohol.

Fermentation A chemical process of breakdown of complex substances by ferments and yeasts combining with oxygen, normally involving yeasts, bacterial and moulds; eg glucose and acetic acid transform into citric acid.

Free radicals Depriving body of active oxygen, they destroy otherwise healthy cells; linked with aging.

Gluconic acid A sugar acid produced by bacteria. When broken down forms caprylic acid which, with butyric acid (see Glucoronic) can counter candidiasis.

Glucuronic acid The liver's principal detoxifying agent, of particular importance in Kombucha, especially for toxic oil products. Transforms into hyaluronic acid/ glucosamines, essential for collagen, cartilage & sinovial (joint) fluid.

Glucosamines (see polysaccharides)

Haemoglobin Red iron-rich cells in the blood which carry oxygen.

Holistic Term used to note an attitude of recognising the interconnected-ness of all life.

Holistic medicine Takes into account all aspects of patient, including psychological and spiritual predispositions, family and work environments.

Iatrogenic Disorders or illnesses caused by the side effects of conventional medications.

Immune deficiency A state of disequilibrium or dysbiosis when the body's ability to fight disease has been compromised by a wide range of physical and emotional factors, but chiefly through chemical pollution and poor nutrition.

Immune system   The body's defensive system against infection or viral attack with formation of antibodies located in the lymph glands and the blood.

Lactic acid   1: Lactate is produced by bacteria through fermentation. In the liver it creates starch and glycogen for energy. 2: L+lactic acid is essential for digestion and forms lactobacillus, the most helpful substance for food assimilation

Liproprotein   The blood proteins which transport cholesterol required for cell membranes and steroid hormones

Macrophages   White blood cells with the specific ability to ingest bacteria.

Malic acid   An oxygen carrier which assists the liver to detoxify.

Metabolism   The term used for the physical, chemical and energy interaction and interconnectedness throughout the body *Metabolism is the complete range of biochemical processes that take place in our bodies and which produce energy. One measure of health is when our metabolism is in balance, and all our organs are in harmony.

Metastases   Process by which cancerous cells travel through the body to form secondary tumours by blood and lymph channels.

Multiple Sclerosis (MS)   Damage to the sheath surrounding nerve fibres and the subsequent atrophy of the nerves.

Naturopathic   A general term for those medical and health approaches which work with Nature. Also a specific practice.

Nucleic acids   The acids responsible for the genetic code.

Oedema   Swelling caused by fluid retention.

Organic acid   An acid containing a carbon compound

Papaya   The leaves of the paw paw plant are regarded as a powerful remedy and preventative for cancer in Polynesia.

Pathogenic   Disease-causing.

Peptic cells   The protein cells which compose the walls of the stomach.

pH   (potential of hydrogen) measures degree of acidity/alkalinity; 0.1 -6·9 is acid; 7·1 -14 is alkaline (0·1 is most acid, 14 least acid).

Pleomorphism   Enderlein's theory of `several-formedness' which holds that microbiological life goes through cycles from virus through bacteria to fungi, their balance depending on environmental factors.

Polysaccharides   Sugars which form the connective tissue of the organs and which play a part in disposal of metabolic wastes; recent research shows their importance in encouraging macrophages and T-cells (qv).

Probiotics   Working with the microbiological life, eg in Kombucha therapy, assisting the beneficial intestinal flora (*cf* antibiotics).

Prophylactic   Preventative measures to ward off a disease, or for preventative strategy.

RNA   is a nucleic acid which gives the body cells their working instructions.

Symbiosis   Mutual dependence. One substance (eg bacterium) needs (an)others to perform its role effectively.

Synovial Fluid   Keeps the joints lubricated. When this is affected, inflammation of the joints sets in, causing arthritis.

T-cells   An important part of the immune system, they quality control the antibodies that are being made and reject pathogenic material.

Topical Use   Dabbing a pad (cottonwool) soaked in Kombucha liquid directly to the skin.

Usnic acid   An antibiotic sometimes found in the Kombucha beverage.

Virus   The smallest living entity, responsible for most infectious diseases; composed of nucleic acids (*qv*) they are immune to chemical destruction, but controlled by the body's antibodies.

Yeast   Single-celled round fungi reproduce by budding or cell division. Some produce spores (the Kombucha yeasts don't).

RECOMMENDED READING

Ball, John, *Understanding Disease: A Health Practitioner's Handbook*, Daniel, 1994.

Bamforth, Nick, *Trusting the Healer Within*, Amethyst, 1989.

Bamforth, Nick, *ME and the Healer Within*, Amethyst, 1993.

Brogdale Apple & Pear Recipe Book, The, Geerings, *1996.*

Brohn, Penny, *The Bristol Programme*, Century, 1987.

Button, John, *How to be Green*, Century, 1989.

Chaitow, Leon, *Candida Albicans*, Thorsons, 1995.

Cooper, Jean, *Food - Your Miracle Medicine: How to Promote & Treat over 100 Symptoms and Problems*, Simon & Schuster, 1994.

Cooper, Diana, *Light up Your Life*, Ashgrove

Cowan, David & Girdlestone, Rodney, *Safe as Houses?: Ill Health and Electro-stress in the Home*, Gateway, 1996.

Cutland, Liz, *Freedom from the Bottle*, Gateway, 1990.

Daniel, Rosy, *Healing Foods*, Thorsons,

Daniel, Rosy, & Goodman, Sandra, *Cancer and Nutrition, the Positive Evidence*, Bristol Cancer Help Centre

Davies, Jill, *Self-Heal: Home Guide to Herbalism and Natural Healing*, Gateway, 1998.

Davies, S, & Stewart, A., *Nutritional Medicine: The Drug-free Guide to Better Family Health*, Pan 1987.

Dickson, Anne, *A Woman in in Your Own Right,*

Fasching, Rosina, *Tea Fungus Kombucha: The Natural Remedy and its Significance in Cases of Cancer and other Metabolic Diseases*, Ennsthaler, 1987.

Frank, Günther, *Kombucha - Healthy Beverage and Natural Remedy from the Far East*, Ennsthaler, 1995.

Hahn, Tich Nhat, *Be Still and Know: Meditations for Peacemakers*, Rider.

Hall, Nicola, *Reflexology*, Gateway, 1991.

Hamlyn, Ted, *The Healing Art of Homoeopathy*, Keats .

Hay, Louise, *You Can Heal Your Life*, Eden Grove, 1987.

Ho, Dr Mae-Wan, *Genetic Engineering, Dream or Nightmare?*, Gateway, 1998.

Hudson, Clare Maxwell, *The Complete Book of Massage*, Dorling Kindersley

Kenton, Leslie, *The Biogenic Diet*, Century, 1986.

Kenton, Leslie, *Passage to Power*, Century

Kenton, Leslie, *Raw Energy*, Century, 1984.

Kroon, Coen van der, *The Golden Fountain: The Complete Guide to Urine Therapy*, Gateway, 1995.

LeShan, Lawrence, *Cancer as a Turning Point*, Gateway, 1990.

Levine, Stephen, *A Gradual Awakening*, Gateway 1990.

Macbeth, Jessica, *Moon Over Water: Meditation Made Clear, with Techniques for Beginners and Initiates*, Gateway, 1990.

MacManaway, Bruce & Turcan, Johanna, *Healing, the Energy that can Restore Health*, Thorsons, 1983.

McAll, Dr Kenneth, *Healing the Family Tree*, Sheldon, 1982.

Needes, Robin, *You Don't Have to Feel Unwell: Nutrition, Lifestyle, Herbs and Homoeopathy, A Home Guide*, Gateway, 1994.

Northrup, Christine, *Women's Bodies, Women's Wisdom: Creating Physical & Emotional Health*, Bantam, 1994.

Odds, *Candida and Candidiasis*, Ballière Tindall, 1995.

Peale, Norman Vincent, *The Power of Positive Thinking*,

Peer, MarisA, *Forever Young*, Michael Joseph

Readers Digest: Family Health Guide, Readers Digest, 1972.

Schneider, Meir, *Self-Healing: My Life and Vision*, Arkana, 1989.

Schneider, Meir, *The Handbook of Self-Healing*, Arkana, 1997.

Scott Peck, M., *The Road Less Travelled*, Rider, 1983.

Shattock, Ernest H., *Mind Your Body: A Practical Method of Self-Healing*, Turnstone, 1979.

Shattock, Ernest H., *A Manual of Self-Healing*, Turnstone, 1982.

Shapiro, Debbie, *Your Body Speaks Your Mind*, Piatkus, 1992 .

Siegel, Bernie, *Love, Medicine and Miracles*, Rider, 1986.

Strickland, S., *The Organic Garden*, Hamlyn.

Templemore, Vernon, *Let's Get the Fear out of Cancer*, Gateway, 1991.

Tietze, Harald, *Kombucha - Miracle Fungus: The Essential Handbook*, Gateway, 1994.

Tompkins, Peter & Bird, Christopher, *The Secret Life of Plants,*

Upton, Carl, *Psionic Medicine*, Routledge 1974, Element 1983.

Weiner, Michael, *Reducing the Risk of Alzheimers*, Gateway, 1989.

BIBLIOGRAPHY OF KOMBUCHA RESEARCH

Abadie, M., "Association de *Candida mycoderma Reess Lodder et d'Acetobacter xylinum Brown* dans la fermentation des infusion de thé": *Ann.Sc.Nat.Bot.*, no.12, pp.765-80, 1961.

Abele, Johann, "Teepilz Kombucha bei Diabetes?" (Kombucha Mushroom for Diabetes?): *Ner N aturarzt*. 110, no.12, p.31, 1988.

Anon, "About Kombucha": *Sudentendeutche Apothekerzig*, no.38, pp.317-8, 1927.

Anon, Fragkasten-Anfrage: *Die Umschau*, no.31:50, 2 Bilagenseite, 1927.

Anon, "Prohibition of the Japanese mushroom 'Kombucha': *Sudentendeutche Apothekerzig*, no.9:2, p.4, 1928.

Anon, "Advertising the Japanese Mushroom Kombucha and its Preparations": *Sudentendeutche Apothekerzig*, no.9:11, p.105, 1928.

Anon, "The Kombucha Question": *Sudentendeutche Apothekerzig*, no.9:10, pp.95-6, 1928.

Anon, "Kombucha drink, questions & answers": *Dtsch.Esssigindustrie*, no.32:38, pp.333-4, 1928.

Anon, "Effects of the Indian Tea Mushroom": *Droisten Zeit,*, no.54:52, pp.1499-500, Leipzig, 1928.

Anon, "Kombucha, the Miracle Mushroom, Japanese tea mushroom" in *Der Grosse Brockhaus*, vol.10, p.346, Brockhaus, Leipzig, 1931.

Anon, "Tea beer: A new use for tea": *Tea & Coffee Trade Jour.*, Aug, pp.180-2, New York, 1932.

Anon, "Tea-Cider. A new drink in Java": *Tea Q'tly*, no.5, pp.126-7, Ceylon, 1932.

Anon, Alg.Landbouwweekbli.v.: *Nederlandsch-Indie*, no.16:46, pp.1223-5, 1932.

Anon, "Theebier"; Mooie perspectieven vor groot binnen-v.": *Nederlandsch-Indie*, no.16:48, pp.1280-1, 1932.

Anon, "Kombucha", in *Der Grosse Brockhaus*, vol.16, p.498, Brockhaus, Weisbaden, 1955.

Anon, Scientific Research at Nat.Hist.Mus. *Trust.Brit.Mus.*, no.31, p,46, London, 1956.

Anon, "Tea fungus" in *Handbook of indigenous fermented food*, K.H.Steinkraus (ed), p.421, Dekker, New York 1983.

Arauner, A., "Der japanische Teepilz" (The Japanese Tea Mushroom): *Deutsch Essigindustrie*, 33:1, pp.11-12, 1929.

Bacinskaya, A.A., "Morfologij i biologij *bacterium xylinium brown*" (The Morphology and Biology of *Bacterium xylinum Brown*": *Russkij Vrae*, 10:51, pp.2104-8, St.Petersburg 1911.

Bacinskaya, A.A., " O tak' naz'ivaemom manezursco-japonskom gribe i cajnom kvase" (The so-called Manchurian-Japanese Mushroom and Tee-Kvass): *Vracebnaja Gazeta*, 20:30, pp.1063-4, 1913.

Bacinskaya, A.A., "O rasprostranenii 'cajnago kwasa' i *bacterium xylinum brown*" (The Spread of 'Tee-Kvass' and *Bacterium xylinum Brown*): *Zurnal mikrobiologii*, no.1, pp.73-85, Petrograd, 1914.

Barbancik, G.F., *Cainii grib i ego lecebnye svoistva* (The tea fungus and its therapeutic properties): 54pp, Omskoe oblastnoe kniznoe izdatelstvo, 1958.

Barsha, J., & Hibbert, H., "Studies on reactions relating to carbohydrates and polysaccharides. Structure of the cellulose synthesised by the action of *acetobacter xylinus* on fructose and glycerol": *Canad.J.Res*, no.10, pp.170-9, 1934.

Bazarewski, S., "Uberden sogenannten 'Wunderpilz' in den baltischen Provinzen" (Concerning the so-called Miracle Mushroom in the Baltic Province): *Korrblatt Naturforsch-Vereins Riga* no.57, pp.61-80, Riga 1915.

Benk, E., "Uber Teepliz-Getrank": *AID-Verbraucherdienst*, no.33, pp.213-4, 1988.

Bernhauer, K. "The biochemistry of the vinegar bacteria": *Erg.Enzymforschg*. no.7, pp.246-80, 1938.

Begold, M., "Teepliz 'Mo-Gu'": *Waischenfelder Apotheke*, Waischenfeld, Franconia.

Bing, M., "Heilwirkung des 'Kombuschaschwammes" (Health Effects of the Kombucha Mushroom): *Die Umschau*, 32:45, pp.913-4, 1928.

Bing, M., "Der Symbionts *Bacterium xylinum - Schizosaccharomyces Pombe* als Therapeutikum" (The Symbionts *Bacterium xylinum* and *Schizosaccharomyces Pombe* as medicinal agents): *Die medizinische Welt*, 2:42, pp.1575-7, 1928.

Bing, M., "Zur Kombuchafrage" (About the Kombucha Question): *Die Umschau*, 33:6, pp.118-9, 1929.

Blanc, P.J., "Characterization of the tea fungus metabolites": *Biotechnology Letters*, vol.18, no.2, pp.139-42, 1995.

Brehmer, Dr.W.von, *Siphonospora polymorpha*, Link, Haag.

Brown, A.J., "Note on the Cellulose formed by *Bacterium Xylinum*": *J.Chem.Soc.Trans.*, no.51, p.643, 1887.

Brown, A.J., "On an Acetic Ferment which forms Cellulose": *J.Chem.Soc.Trans.*, no.49, pp.432-9, 1896.

Brucker, M.O., "Antwort auf Leseranfrage 'Wundermittel Kombucha?'": *Natur i.heilen*, no.65, p.536. 1988.

Brucker, M.O., "Antwort auf Leseranfrage zu Kombucha": *Der Naturarzt*, no.108, p.14, 1986.

Buu-Hoi, N.P., & Ratsimamanga, A.R. "Kojic acid, active principle in the *Aspergillus flavus oryzea* culture": *C.R.Acad.Sci.* no.286, pp.341-3, Paris 1953.

Caesar, W., "Von kombu zu kombucha": *Deutsche Apotheker Zet.* no.130, p.2267, 1990.

Chambionnat, M., "Contrbution a l'etude du champignon japonais": *Bull.Soc.Hist.Nat.Maroc*, no.33, pp.3-8, 1952.

Dahl, J., "Ein Glas Pilz - ohne Schaum": *Natur*, no.7, pp.73-4, 1987.

Danielova, L.T., "Bakteriostaticeskoe i baktericidnoe svoistvo nastoia 'cainogo griba'" (The bacteriostatic and bactericidal properties of the 'tea-fungus' infusion) *Trudy Yerevanskogo zoovet.Inst.*, no.11, pp.31-41, 1949.

Danielova, L.T., "K morfologii 'cainogo griba'" (The Morphology of the 'tea fungus'): *Trudy Yerevanskogo zoovet.Inst.*, no.17, pp.201-16, 1954.

Danielova, L.T., "Biologiceskie osobennosti cainogo griba" (The special biological characteristics of the tea fungus): *Trudy Yerevanskogo zoovet.Inst.*, no.23, pp.159-64, 1959.

Danielova, L.T., "Cainii grib *medusomyces gisevii*" (The 'tea fungus' *medusomyces gisevii*), doctoral dissert. at Moskova Vet.Acad., 36pp, 1954.

Danielova, L.T. & Sakaryan, G.A., *Teyi saki koultouran ew nra kiraroume anasnapahoutyan mej Yerevan: gitoutyan glavor varcoutyan hratarkcoutyoun* (The tea kvass culture and its use in stockbreeding): Min.of Agric, 160pp, Yerevan 1959.

Dalielova, L.T., "Biolgiceskie osobennost cajnogo griba": *Trudy Erevanskogo zoovet.Inst*, no.23, pp.159-64, 1959.

Dinslage, E. & Ludorff, W., "Der 'indische Teepilz'" (The Indian tea-mushroom): *Z.Unters.Lebensmittel*, no.53, pp.458-67, 1927.

Dubowitz, H., "Der japanische Pilz" (The Japanese Mushroom): *Gyogyaszai*, no.67:12, pp.274-5, Budapest, 1927.

Dutton, G.J. (ed), *Glucuronic Acid*: Academic Press, 1966.

Dutton, G.J., *Glucuronidation of Drugs and Other Compounds*: CRC Press, 1980.

Eberding, W., "The Japanese Tea Mushroom": *Volksheil* 5:5, pp.123-4, Berlin 1928.

Enderlein, Prof.Dr.Gunter, *Akmon*, vol.1, nos.1- 1955, 2- 1957 & 3- 1959, Ibica, Aumuhle/Hamburg.

Fasching, R., *Tea Fungus Kombucha: The Natural Remedy and its Significance in Cases of Cancer and other Metabolic Diseases*: Ennsthaler, Steyr, 1987.

Fasching, R., "Krebs heilen mit dem Teepilz Kombucha" (Cancer cured with the Kombucha tea fungus): *Diagnosen*, no.8, pp.62-5, 1986.

Fasching, R., "Pilz gegen Pilz": *Diagnosen*, no.8, pp.64-6, 1988.

Fedorow, M.V., "Mikrobiologija": *Gos.izdatel'stvo sel'skohoz.lit.*, Moskva, no.236, 1949.

Filho, L.X., Paulo, M.Q., Pareira, E.C. & Vicente, C. "Phenolics from tea fungus analysed by high performance liquid chromatography": *Phyton*, vol.45, no.2, pp.187-191, Buenos Aires, 1985.

Floresco, N., "Tadpoles Nourished by Kombucha": *Bull.Fac.Stiinte Cernautl*, 4:1, pp.157-8, (Romanian) 1930.

Floresco, N., "Kombucha, A Psychological Study": *Bull.Fac.Stiinte Cernautl*, 4:1, pp.146-156, (Romanian) 1930.

Floresco, N., & Rafailesco-Floresco, A., "Kombucha: Influence on the Development of Frog Eggs": *Bull.Fac.Stiinte Cernautl*, 4:1, pp.159-163, (Romanian) 1930.

Floresco, N., "Kombucha, Influence on the Development of the Tadpole": *Bull.Fac.Stiinte Cernautl*, 4:2, pp.220-6, (Romanian) 1930.

Floresco, N., "Kombucha, Influence on the Isolated Heart": *Bull.Fac.Stiinte Cernautl*, 4:1, pp.252-4, (Romanian) 1930.

Floresco, N., "Kombucha: Ferment Solubles": *Bull.Fac.Stiinte Cernautl*, 5:1, pp.1-14, (Romanian) 1931.

Fluck, V. & Steinegger, E., "Things worth knowing about the tea mushroom" (see: Steiger & Steinegger, "The Tea Mushroom: *Osterr.Apoth.Zig.*, no.11:47, pp.580-3, 1957.

Fluck, V. & Steinegger, E., "Eine neue Hefekomponente des Teeplizes": *Scientia Pharmaceutica*, no.25, pp.43-4, Vienna, 1957.

Frank, N., "The clinical value of an oral antidiabetic medicine" (*see* Gutmann, C.): *Chem.Zbl.*, vol.I, p.1489, Vienna, 1930.

Frank, G. W., *Heilkrafte der Natur aus einem Pilz - Der Teepliz Kombucha*: Birkenfeld, 44pp., 1988.

Frank, G.W., "Kombucha (Antwort auf Leseranfrage)": *Sonnseitig leben*, 40:241, Zurich, 1989.

Frank, R., "Zuckerproblem beim Kombucha-Tee (Antwort auf Leseranfrage)": *Natur & Heilen*, Munchen, no.65, pp.298-9, 1988.

Funke, Hans, "Der Teepilz Kombucha" (The Kombucha tea fungus): *Natur & Heilen* no.64, pp.509-13, 1987.

Gadd, C.H., "Tea Cider": *Tea Qu'tly*, no.6, pp.48-53, Ceylon, 1933.

Gince, V. "Japnoski grobok": *Gigiena Pitanija*, vol.1, p.15, Leningrad, 1928.

Glas, Gerhard, "Wie wird das Kombucha-Getrank angesetzt?": *Kurier*, no.19, p.89, 1987.

Gordienko, M., see Utkin, L. "A new micro-organism from the group of vinegar bacteria": *Zbl.Bakt*, 98:II, p.359, 1937.

Golz, H., *Kombucha - Ein altes Teeheilmittel schenkt neue Gesundheit*, 4ed: Ariston, Genf, 1992.

Gotz, Georg, "Kombucha - der Wunderpilz, der Millionen Gesundheit schenkt": *Das Neue*, nos.3-14, Bauer, Hamburg, 1988.

Gutmann, C. & Kallfelz, H, "The clinical value of an oral antidiabetic medicine": *Klin.Woehenschr.* vol.8, pp.2246-7, (German) 1929.

Haehn, H, & Engel, M., "Uber die Bildung von Milchsaure durch *Bacterium xylinum*. Milchsauregarung durch Kombucha" (The Synthesis of Lactic Acid by *Bacterium xylinum*. Lactic acid fermentation by Kombucha): *Z.Bakt.Parasitenkde/Infektionskrahkh*, vol.79, pp.182-5, 1929.

Hahmann, C., "Uber Drogen und Drogenverfalschungen": *Apotheker-Zeit.*, vol.44, no.37, pp.561-3, 1929.

Hansel, R., & Schimmitat, I., "Was ist wirklich dran am Kombucha-Pilz?": *Arztliche Praxis*, no.12, pp.1704-5, 1989.

Harms, H., "Der japanisch Teepliz" (The Japanese Tea Mushroom): *Therapeut.Berichte*, no.12, pp.498-500, 1927.

Harms, H., "The Japanese or Indian Tea Mushroom": *Xrztlicher Wegweiser*, 4:17, p.330, Berlin 1928.

Harms, H., "The Japanese Tea Mushroom": *Pharm.Ber.*, 3:1, pp.1-3, (German) 1928.

Harms, H., "The Tea Mushroom, Mo-Gu": *Chem.Zbl.*, vol.11, p.602, (German) 1929.

Harms, H., "Health effects of the 'Kombucha mushroon'": *Die Umschau*, no.32 (45), pp.913-4, 1928.

Harnish, G., *Kombucha -gebalte Heilkraft aus der Natur*: Bietigheim-Bissingen, Turm, 1991.

Hauser, S.P., "Dr.Sklenar's Kombucha Mushroom Infusion - a Biological Cancer Therapy": *Schweiz Runsch.Med.Prax.*, no.79, pp.243-6, 1990.

Henneberg, W., "Spezielle Pilzkunde, unter besonderer Berucksichtigung der Hefe-, Essig- und Milchsaurebakterien", in *Handbuch der Garungsbakteriologie* (Handbook of Fermentative Bacteriology): vol.2, pp.70,225,379, Parey, Berlin, 1926.

Hennenberg, W., "Zur Kenntnis der Schnellessig und Weinessigbakterien": *Zentralbaltt fur Bakteriologie*, vol.19, no.25, pp.789-804, 1907.

Hensler, P.O., "Alles uber Kombucha" (All about Kombucha): Stutensee, 1989.

Hermann, S., "Die sogenannte 'Kombucha'" (Kombucha is what it's called): *Umschau*, no.22, pp.841-4, 1929.

Hermann, S., "Uber die sogenannte Kombucha" (Concerning what is called Kombucha): *Biochem.Zeit*. no.192, pp.176-99, 1928.

Hermann, S.,"The synthesis of gluconic acid and ketogluconic acid by *Bacterium gluconicum, bacterium xylinum* and *bacterium xylinoides*", *Biochem.Z.*, vol.214, pp. 357-67, (German) 1929.

Hermann, S., "Pharmacological investigations of the so-called Kombucha and its influence on the toxic effects of Cholecalciferol": *Klin.Wochenschr.*,vol.8, pp.1752-7, (German) 1929.

Hermann, S.,"Zur Pharamkologie der Gluconsaure" (The pharamcology of gluconic acid. A contribution to the problem of the effects of free acids in the organism): *Naunyn-Schmiedebergs Arch.exp.Pathol-Pharm.*, vol.154, pt.I, pp.43-81; pt.II 141-160; pt.III pp.179-192, 1930.

Hermann, S., & Fodor, N., "C-Vitamin - (l-Ascorbinsaure) - Bildung durch eine Symbiose von Essigbakterien und Hefen" (Vitamin C production from a symbiosis of vinegar bacteria and yeats: *Biochem.Z.* no.276 5:6, pp.323-5, 1935.

Hermann, S. & Neuschul, P., "The biochemistry of vinegar bacteria and a proposal for a new systematic treatment": *Biochem.Z.* no.283, pp.129-216. (German) 1931.

Hermann, S. & Neuschul, P., "Lactic and pyruvic acid synthesis from vinegar bacteria": *Biochem.Z.* 4:6, pp.446-59, (German) 1931.

Hermann, S. & Neuschul, P.,"The biochemistry of vinegar bacteria. A characteristic difference of bactrium gluconicum from other vinegar bacteria concerning the influence of glactose": *Biochem.Z.* no.270, 1:3, pp.6-14, (German) 1934.

Hermann, S. & Neuschul, P., "The oxidation of glucose from *bacterium gluconicum hermann*": *Biochem.Z.* no.287 5:6, pp.400-4, (German) 1936.

Hesseltine, C.W., "A Millennium of Fungi, Food & Fermentation": *Mycologia*, no.57, pp.149-197, New York 1965.

Hesseltine, C.W., "Industrial Mycology, tea fungus": Mycolgica, no.57, pp.177-9, 1965.

Heubner, W., *Otto Heubners Lebenschronik* (Otto Heubner's Lifestories), no.228, Springer, Berlin, 1927.

Hobbs, Christopher, *Kombucha: Tea Mushroom - The Essential Guide:* Botanica Press, 1995.

Irion, H., "Fungus japonicus, Fungojapon Kombucha - Indisch-japanischer Teepilz": *Lehrgang fur Drogistenfachschulen*, vol.2, Muller, Berlin-Leipsig, 1944.

Irion, H., (ed), *Lehrgang fur Droistenfrachschule in 4 Bänden*, (Botany, vol.2 - Lore of Drugs, p.405): Muller, Eberswalde-Berlin-Leipzig, 1942.

Kaminski, A., "Arzte: Pilz heilt Frauenleiden" (*Bild der Frau*, no.2), Springer, Hamburg, 1988.

Kasevnik, L.D., "Biochimija Vit.C. Soobscenie III. O sposobnosti Japonskogo cajnogo griba sintezirovat Vit.C" (The biochemistry of Vitamin C: Ability of the Japanese tea mushroom to sythesize vit.C): *Bull.exp.Biol.i Med*, no.3 (1), Moscow 1937.

Kasevnik, L.D., "O Nekotorii biohimiceskii osobennostia t.n. 'cainogo griba'" (Some special biochemical characteristics of the co-called 'tea fungus'): *Sborinik trudov Archangelskii gosudarstvennii mediciniskii Inst.*, no.5, pp.116-21.

Kasevnik, L.D., "A biochemical peculiarity of the so-called tea mushroom" *Medicinskij Inst.*, no.5, pp.116-21, (Russian) 1940.

Kasevnik, L.D., Pyumima, V.I. & Nebolyubova, G.E., "Materialy k biohimii tak naz. 'Cainogo griba'. Soobscenie IV: O bakteriostaticeskom deistvii ekstrakta iz nastioia 'Cainogo griba'" (Contributions to the biochemistry of the so-called 'tea fungus'. Report IV:

The bacteriostatic powers of the extract of the 'tea fungus' infusion): *Trudy Tomskogo medicinskogo Inst.*, no.13, pp.115-7.

Kobert, K. *Der Kvass - ein unschadliches billiges Volksgetsrank* (The Kwass - a harmless, low cost people's drink), 82pp, Tausch & Grosse, 1913.

Kobert, R., "About Kvass: Its Introduction into Western Europe": *Hist.Stud.Pharm.*, Inst.Univ.Dorpat, no.5, pp.100-131, (German) 1896.

Kobert, R., "Tea Kvass": *Mikrokosmos*, 11:9, p.159, (German) 1917.

Kohler, V., "Glukuronsaure macht Krebspatiente Mut" (Glucuronic acid gives cance patients hope): *Arzlichte Praxis*, no.33, p.887, 1981.

Kohler, V. & Kohler, J., "Glukuronsaure als okologische Hilfe" (Glucuronic acid as an ecological aid): in *Sofortheilung des Waldes*, vol.1 (ed. Kaegelmann), Windeke-Rosbach, 1985.

Konovalov, I.N., Litvinov, M.A. & Zakman, L.M., "Izmenenie prirody i fiziologiceskii osobennostei cainogo griba medusomyces gisevii lindau v zavisimosti ot uslovii kultivirovania" (Changes in the nature and psysiological properties of the tea fungus medusomyces gisevii lindau regarding the requirments of the culture medium): *Bot Zurnal*, vol.44, no.3, pp.346-9, Moscow 1959.

Konovalov, I.N. & Semenova, M.N., "The physiology of the tea mushroom" *Bot.Zurnal*, no.40, pp.567-70, Moscow 1955.

Koolhaus, D.R., "Tea Beer": *Alg.Landboiuwweekbl.* 16:48, p.1295, (Dutch) 1931.

Koolhaus, D.R., & Boedijn, K.B., "The tea-mushroom": *De Bergcultures* no.6, pp.259-60, Djakarta 1932.

Koolhaus, D.R., & Boedijn, K.B., "De 'Tea Mushroom' in Nederlandsh-Indie, Vorooplige Mededeeling" (The tea-mushroom in the Dutch East Indies): *De Bergcultures* no.6, pp.299-303, 1932.

Korner, H., "Der Teepilz Kombucha" (The tea fungus Kombucha): *Der Naturarzt*, vol.108, no.5, pp.14-6, 1987.

Korner, H., "Kombucha-Zubereitung wurde von Sportmedizinern getestet" (Kombucha preparation tested by sports physicians): *Natura-med*, vol.4, no.10, p.592, 1989.

Korner, H., "Die Heilkraft des Pilzes Kombucha": *Raum & Zeit*, no.20, 1986.

Korner, H., "Ein Parasit im Blut" (A parasite in the blood): *Raum & Zeit*, no.19, 1985.

Korner, H., "Kombucha - wertvolles Geschenk der Natur": *Naturheilpraxis*, no.39, 1986.

Kozacki, M., Koizumi, A. & Kotahara, K., "Microorganism of Zoogleal Mats formed in Tea Decoction": *Jour.Food Hyg.Soc.Japan*, no.13, pp.89-96, 1972.

Kraft, M.-M., "Le Champignon de The" (The tea mushroom): *Nova Hedwigia*, no.1, pp.297-304, 1959.

Kreger-van Rij, N.J.W. (ed), *The Yeasts - A Taxonomic Study*, 3ed, Amsterdam, Elsevier Science, 1987.

Lakowitz, N., "Teepilz und Teekwass" (The Tea Mushroom and Tea Kvass): *Apoth.Zeit.*, 43:19, pp.298-300, 1928.

Lakowitz, N., "Teekwass": *Der Naturforscher*, 5:1, pp.18-9, (German) 1929.

Lederer, N., "The Japanese Mushroom": *Biolog.Heilkunst*, no.8, p.579, (German) 1927.

Leskov, A.I., "Novye svedenya o cainom gribe" (New information about the tea fungus): *Feldser i Akuerka*, vol.23, no,10, pp.47-8, Moscow, 1958.

Lind, J., "En ganske ny Form af Medicin" (A new form of Medicine): *Arch.Pharm/Chemi.*, no.32, p.336, Kobenhavn 1926.

Lindau, G., "Uber *Medusomyces gisevii*, eine neue Gattung und Art der Hefewpilze" (Concerning *Medusomyces gisevii*, a new genus and species of yeast mushroom), *Ber.dt.bot.Ges.*, no.31, pp.243-8, 1913.

Lindner. P., "Die vermeintliche neue Hefe *medusomycs gisevii*", *Ber.dt.bot.Ges.*, no.32, pp.364-8, 1913.

Lindner, P., Uber Teekwass und Teekwasspilze", *Mikrokosmos*, no.11, pp.93-8, 1917.

Lindner, P. "Tea Kvass and the Tea Kvass Mushroom": *Deutsch Essigindustrie*, 22, pp.273-4, 278-80, 284-5, (German) 1918.

List, P.H., Hufschmidt, W., "Basische Pilzinhaltsstoffe. 5. Mitteilung uber biogene Aminine und Aminosauren des Teepilzes": *Phar.Zentrtalhalle*, no.98, pp.593-8, 1959.

Lowenheim, H., "Uber den induischen Teepilz" (The Indian Tea Mushroom): *Apoth.Zeit.*, vol.42, pp.148-9, 1927.

Madaus, in *Biolog.Heilkunst*, no.15, 1929, quoted by Arauner, 1929.

Mann, U., "Verbluffend - ein Pilz kuriert den Darm.Bild. und Funk" (Amazing - a mushroom that heals the intestines): *Bild und Funk*, no.35, Burda, Offenburg, 1988.

Matern, S, Bock, K.W. & Gerok, W. (eds.), *Advances in Glucoronic Conjugation*: MTP Press, Lancaster, 1985.

Martell, P., "The Tea Mushroom as a Medicine": *Pharm.Zentralhalle*, vol.70, pp.614-8, (German) 1929.

Matouschek, F. "The so-called 'Miraculous Mushroom' in the Baltic Province": *Zbl.Bakteriol.*, II:55, pp.320-1 (Russia) 1922.

Mayser, P., Fromme, S., Leitzmann, C. & Grunder, K., "The yeast spectrum of the 'tea fungus Kombucha'": *Mycoses*, no.38, pp.289-95, 1955.

Meixner, A., *Pilzer selber zuchten* (Cutivating mushrooms yourself): 96pp, Aarau, 1989.

Meixner, A., "Combucha, der Teepilz": *Sudwestdeutsche Piz-Rundschau*, no.2, pp.1-4, 1983.

Merk Index, "Glucuronic Acid", p.701; "Usnic Acid", p.1557, 11th ed. 1989.

Molitor, H., "Which position should doctors take on the Kombucha question?" (see Wiechowski, W.: *Die Taglicke Praxis*, 1:2, pp.43-4, Wien 1929.

Mollenda, L. "Kombucha, ihre Heilbedeutung und Zuchtung" (Kombucha, its significance for health and cultivation): *Deutsch Essigindustrie*, 32:27, pp.243-4, 1928.

Muhietaler, K. "The structure of bacterial cellulose": *Biochim.et Biophys.* Acta 8, pp.527-35, (German) 1949.

Mulder, D., "A revival of tea cider": *Tea Qu'tly* , Ceylon, no.32, pp.48-53, 1961

Mullerova, L., "Kombucha": *Casopis Ceskovslovenskeho Lekarnietva* 7:4, pp.58-9, (Czech) 1927.

Mullerova, N., "Japanese Houba": *Prakticky Lekar*, 7:3, p.119 (Czech) 1927.

Naumova. E.K., "Meduzin - Novoe antibiioticeskoe vescestvo, obrazumoe *Medusmyces gisevii*, Vtoraya naucnaya Konferencia sasitarnogigieniceskogo fakulteta: (Medusin - a new antibiotic substance formed by *Medusomyces gisevii* in 2nd Scientific Conference of the Faculty of Health & Hygiene": *Kazanskii Gosudarstvfenni Med.Inst.*, pp.20-3, (Russian) 1949.

Obst, W., "Banana Vinegar and the Tea Mushroom": *Deutsch Essigindustrie*, 33:18, pp.145-6, (German) 1929.

Pascal, Alana *with* Van der Kar, Lynne, *Kombucha: How-To and What's it all About:* Van der Kar Press, 1995.

Paula Gomes, A. de, "Observacoes sobre a utilzacao de Zymomonas mobilis (Lindner), Kluyver et van Nierl, 1936: *Revista Inst.de Antibioticos*, Parnambuco, Brasil, no.1, pp.77-81, 1959.

Popiel, L. von, "Zur Selbstherstellung von Essig" (On making vinegar yourself): *Pharmaz.Post*, vol.50, no.80, pp.757-8, Vienna 1917.

Pletnitzky, A., *Ars Medici*, no.17, p.604, Vienna 1927.

Prod'hom, G., "Mushroom of charity": *Bull.romand. Mucolog.*, Dec.1955, Lausanne 1955.

Propfe, P., "Kombucha": *Die Umschau*, 33:6, p.118, (German) 1929.

Radu, A. "Ciuperca de ceai" (Tea Mushroom): *Farm.Rev.Soc.Stintelor Med*. no.4 (4) pp.306-13, Bucarest 1956.

Reiss, J., "Der Teepilz und seine Stoffwechselprodukte" (The Tea mushroom and its metabolic components): *Deuts.Lebenmittel-Rundschau*, vol.82, no.9, pp.286-90, 1987.

Reith, H., "Differential-Diagnose de Candida-Pilze": *Arch.f.Klin.und exp.Derm*. no.205, pp.541-50.1958.

Rentz, N. (see: Tindimnik, V.S., Funk, S.E. & Sabinskaja, I.V.), *Chem.Zbl*. II 2489 (Russian) 1951.

Roots. H., "Teeseeneleotise Ravitoimest, Noukogude eest tervishoid" (The curative powers of the tea fungus): no.2, pp.55-7, (Estonian) Tallin, 1959.

Rose, A.H. & Harrison, J.S., *The Yeasts* 2ed, vol.1, Academic, London 1973.

Rosenbaum, J. "Kombucha": *Practicky Lekar*, 7:15, pp.604, Praha 1927.

Rywosch, S., "Kombucha, a New Drink": *Die Umschau*, 32:30, pp.610-4 (German) 1928.

Rywosch, S., "The Japanese Tea Mushroom and Arteriosclerosis": *Dir Weisse Fahne*, 9:4, pp.184-5, (German) 1928.

S., "Der 'japanische Teepliz' - Die Weisse Fahne": *Zeitblatter zur Verinnerlichung Vergeistigung*, no.9, pp.184-5, Wurttemburg, 1928.

Saccardo, P.A., *Medusomuyces Gisevii*, Sylloge Fungorum 24, sec.II, 1314, Coheredum Saccardo, 1485, Avellino (Italian) 1928.

Saito, K., "Technically-important East-Indian Mushrooms": *Mikrocosmos*, 5:7, pp.145-150, 1911.

Sakaryan, G.A. & Danielova, L.T., "Antibioticeskie svoistvga nastoia griba *Medusomyces gisevii* (cainogo griba)" (The antibiotic significance of the liquid substance from *Medusomyces gisevii* [tea mushroom]): *Trud'i Erevanskogo zooveterinarigo Inst*. no.10, pp.33-45, (Russian) 1948.

Sakarjan, G.A. & Danielova, L.T., "Lecebn'ie svojstva cajnogo griba (Medusomyces gisevi)" (The curative power of the tea mushroom): Vetinerarija no.26 (10), pp.48-9, Moskva 1949.

Sass, E.Ju., "O cajnom gribe" (The tea mushroom): *Aptecnoje delo*" no.5, pp.41-2, Moskva, 1952.

Scerbacev, D.M., "Cajn'ij ili japonski grib i ego problema" (The tea mushroom or Japanese mushroom and its transformation): *Sovetskaja Farm*. 5:6, pp.28-9, (Russian) 1931.

Schmidt, I, *Der Teepliz - morphologische, physiologische und therapeutische Untersuchungen* (Dissertation for teaching degree), 51pp, Bochum, 1979.

Schreyer, R., "Comparative investigations of the synthesis of gluconic acid from the 'mould mushroom'": *Biochem.Z.*, no.240, pp.295-325, (German) 1931.

Schroder. H., "Teepilz und japanische Kristalle": *Deine Geseundhiet*, No.7, pp.29-30, Berlin, 1989.

Schroder. H., "Die japanischen Meereskristalle": *Brandenburgisches Neueste Nachrihten*, 8 May, p.6, 1989.

Schwaibold, N., "The biochemistry of vit.C.: The capacity of the Japanese tea mushroom to synthesize vit.C: (see: Kasevnik, L.D) *Chem.Zbl.*, 1937.

Sievers, M., Lanini, C., Weber, A., Schuler-Schmid, U. & Teuber, M., "Microbiology and fermentation balance in Kombucha beverage obtained from a tea fungus fermentation": *Syst.Appl.Microbiol*. Vol18, pp.590-4, Fischer 1995.

Silva, R.L.de & Saravanapavan, T.V., "Tea cider - a potential winner": *Tea Qu'tly*, no.39, pp.37-40, Ceylon, 1969.

Sklenar, R., "Ein in der Iris sichtbarer Test fur eine Stoffwechselstorung, kontrolliert an Hand von Dunkelfelduntersuchungen des Blutes nach Scheller": Erfahrungsheilkunde, no.13, 1964.

Sklenar, Dr.R., *Krebsdiagnose aus dem Blut und die Behandlung von Krebs und Prakanzerosen mit der Kombucha und Kolipraparaten* (Cancer diagnosis through the blood and the treatment of cancer and precancerous ailments by means of Kombucha and colicines): Fasching, Klangenfurt, 1983.

Sklenar, Dr.R., in *Sonderdruck aus Erfahrungsheilkunde. Zeitschrift fur die tagliche Praxis*, vol.XIII, issue.3: Haug, Ulm-Donau, 1964

Stadelmann, E., "Der Teepliz - Eine Literaturzusammenstellung" (The tea mushroom - a compilation of literature): *Sydowia, ann.mycolg.*, ser.2, pp.380-8, 1957.

Stadelmann, E., "Der Teepilz un seine antibiotische Wirkung" (The tea mushroom and its antibacterial action - a bibiliography): *Zentralblatt Bakt.I.Abte.ref.*, no.180, pp.401-35, 1961.

Stadelmann, E., "Die Symbiose Tibi, *Bulletin de la Société Fribourgeoise des Sciences Naturelles*, no.47, pp.16-9, 1957.

Stark, J.B., Walter, E.D. & Owens, H.S., "Method of Isolation of Usnic Acid from Ramalina retuculata": *Jour.Amer.Chem.Soc.*, no.72, pp.1919-20, 1950.

Steinmann, A., "The Indian 'Tea Mould'": *De Bergcultures*, 2:II, pp.1113-4, Djakarta, 1928.

Steiger, K.E. & Steinegger, E. "Uber den Teepilz" (The tea mushroom): *Pharm.Acta Helv.* no.32, pp.86-93, 133-54, (Swiss) 1957.

Strubin, M., "Mushroom of Charity": *Bull.rom.Mucolog.*, Feb.1956.

Subov, M.I. "The significance of tea with the so-called 'tea mushroom' as a therapeutic agent": *Vrac.delo*, no.27 (6), pp.511-2, (Russian) 1947.

Sukiasyan, A.O., "Vliyanie faktorov vnesnei sredy i istocnikov pitanya na nakoplenie antibioticeskii vescestv v kulture 'cainogo griba': Soobscenie 1. Izucenie razlicnii fiziko-mehaniceskii vozodeistvii" (The influence of culture milieu factors and nutrient sources on the accumulation of antibiotic substances in 'tea fungus' cultures. 1st report: the investigation of various physico-mechanical influences): *Trudy Yerevanskogo zoovet.Inst.*, no.17, pp.229-35. 1954.

Tea Export Bureau, Batavia, "Tea cider - a new drink in Java": *Tea Qu'tly*, no.5, pp.126-7, Ceylon, 1932.

Thomas, R.D., "The Nature and Chemical Effects of the Mother of Vinegar": *Ann.Chem.Pharm.*, no.83, pp.89-93, 1852.

Tietze, H., *Kombucha - Miracle Fungus: The Essential Handbook*, Gateway, Bath, 1994.

Tietze, H., *Kombucha, the Miracle Fungus*, Tietze Pubs, Bermagui, 1994.

Tindimnik, V.S., Funk, S.E. & Sabinskaja, I.V., "Kvoprosu o terapevticeskih svojstvah cajnogo griba" (The question of the therapeutic vinegar bacteria quality of the tea mushroom): *Terapevticeskif Archiv*. no.23 (1), pp.85-7, (Russian) 1951.

Utkin, L., "O novom mikroorganizme iz gruppy uksusnyi bakterii" (On a new micro-organism of the acetic acid group): *Mikrobiologia*, vol.6, no.4, pp.421-34, Moscow, 1937.

Valentin, H., "Uber die Verwendung des indsichen Teeplizes und seine Gewinnung in trockener Form" (The Usability of the Indian tea mushroom and its extraction in in dried form): *Apot.Zeit*, no.43, pp.1533-6, 1928.

Valentin, H., "Wesentliche Bestandteile der Garungsprodukte in den durch Pilztatigkeit gewonnenen Hausgetranken sowie die Verbreitung der letzteren" (Primary active components of fermentation products from mushroom-extracted home drinks, as well as its spread): *Apoth.Zeit.*, 45:91, pp.1464-5; 45:92, pp.1477-8, 1930.

Vasilikov, B.P., "O 'Cajnom gribe'" (Tea mushroom): *Priroda*, no.39 (7), pp.59-60, Leningrad 1950.

Waldeck, H., "Der Teepliz" (The Tea Mushroom): Pharm.Zentralhalle, no.68, pp.789-90, 1927.

Weihowski, W., "Welche Stellung soll der Arzt zur Kombuchafrage einnehmen?" (Which position should doctors take on the Kombucha question?) (see: Molitor, H.): *Beitr.arzt.Fortbildg.* 6:1, pp.2-10, Prague 1928.

Yermolayeva, Z.V., Vaisberg, G.E. & Afanaseyva, T.I. & Givenstal, N.I., "O stimulyacii nekotorii antibakterialnii faktorov v organizme zitvotnii" (The stimulation of specific antibacterial factors in the animal organism): *Antibiotiki*, no.3 (6), pp.46-50, Moscow 1958.

Zamkow, N. "Russischer Tee-Essig. Uber den sogenannten mandschurisch-japanischen Pilz und Teekwass" Russian Tea-vinegar: The so-called Manchurian-Japanese mushroom and Tea Kvass): *Deutsch Essigindustrie*, 18:28, pp.330-1, (German), 1914.

Zeller, A.P., *Das Reich der Hausfrau*, Ensslin-Drick, Reutlingen, 1924.

Zimmermann, W. "Wogegen hilft der Kombucha-Pilz?" (Expertenanfrage): *Fortchritte der Medizin*, no.107, p.13, Munich, 1989.

RESOURCE SECTION AND SUPPLIERS

Please enclose an A4 s.a.e. (stamped, self-addressed envelope) when writing for a mail order catalogues and price lists. For overseas enquiries enclose an international postage coupon. Thank you.

MAIL ORDER - KOMBUCHA AND RELATED PRODUCTS

BRITAIN

KOMBUCHA CULTURES/ BOOKS/ INFORMATION /NEWSLETTER: Obtain your own healthy Kombucha starter culture to make Kombucha tea at home, contact: **The Kombucha Tea Network UK,** PO Box 1887, Bath BA2 8YA. The 'Network' has been set up by a team of committed people, each of whom co-ordinates and supplies people in their local area of the country. The cultures are charged for their costs only - of preparation and mailing.

NB Kombucha cultures are not on sale retail in any shops, as they are a 'live' product.

COMMERCIAL BEVERAGE - *Kombuchai:* **Kombucha Pool of Life Ltd** make ready to drink Kombucha in one litre bottles. Made with Japanese Bancha green tea for its health-giving properties. Can be purchased or ordered through your local health food shop.

ELECTRIC HEATING TRAYS/ pH TEST STRIPS/ KOMBUCHA CAPSULES/ GREEN TEA and other related Kombucha products available from: **Kombucha Supplies UK,** The Hollies, Mill Hill, Wellow, Bath BA2 8QJ, Tel: 01225 833 150; Fax: 01225 840 012. Also gives advice on Kombucha brewing - weekday mornings, (Kombucha authors).

AUTHENTIC CONTINUOUS FERMENTATION KOMBUCHA JAR in two sizes (see page 39) available only from: **Harmonic Health**, 36 Braemar Ave., London, N22 7BY. Tel/Fax: 0181 889 1426.

PAW PAW CONCENTRATE and **THE RENE CAISSE FORMULA TEA** (ESSIAC) available from: **Kombucha Supplies UK,** The Hollies, Mill Hill, Wellow, Bath, BA2 8QJ, Tel: 01225 833 150; Fax: 01225 840 012.

Essiac Information Pool is a service which supplies and makes available information on re-quest of the herbal formula; Address - Room for Healing, Inver, Co. Donegal, Rep. of Ireland. Tel: 073 36406.

HERBS: Baldwins stock the largest range in the UK. of herbs, roots, barks, tinctures and fluid extracts; 173 Walworth Rd., London SE17 1RW Tel: 0171 703 5550.

HERBS: Napiers Herbal stock a large range of herbs, tinctures etc. Also has an Apothecary shop in Edinburgh and Glasgow with fully qualified herbal practitioners available for consultation: Forest Bank, Barr, Ayrshire, KA26 9TN, Scotland. Tel: 01465 861 625.

TEAS: quality teas and herbal infusions: **The Tea House,** Covent Garden, 15 Neal St., London, WC2H 9PU. Tel: 0171 240 7539; Fax: 0171 836 4769.

WATER FILTERS: Roger Sanders willingly gives advice on the best filter for your needs: **The Well-Being Research Centre,** Westend Farm, 5 Far St, Wymeswold, Leics. LE12 6TZ. Tel: 01509 880 447.

VORTEX WATER SPIRALISER: To Re-energise all your water contact: **Aquarian Angel Services,** 23 West Mount, Guildford, Surrey, GU2 5HL. Tel/Fax: 01483 572 688.

USA

KOMBUCHA CULTURES: The **Kombucha Foundation** (Kombucha authors) has a data bank for people who require a culture and others offering them: PO Box 661056, Los Angeles, CA 90066.

KOMBUCHA MUSHROOMS / INFORMATION: for further information contact; **Laurel Farms**, Ms Betsy Prior (Kombucha author), PO Box 7405, Studio City, CA 91614.

READY MADE KOMBUCHA BEVERAGE/ KOMBUCHA CULTURES: for further information contact: **Lee Vinocur**, PO Box 81, Palm Springs, CA 92258 Tel/Fax: 619 329 9813.

AQUARIUM HEATERS / pH STRIPS: The Van Der Kar Press, Attn. Mail Order Dept. PO Box 189, Malibu, CA 90265-2855.

AUSTRALIA

KOMBUCHA CULTURES/ HERBS/ GREEN TEAS/ HEATED MATS: Harald Teitze (Kombucha author) PO Box 34, Bermagui South, NSW 2546. Tel: +61 64 934 552; Fax: +61 64 34 900.

READY MADE KOMBUCHA / PAW PAW CONCENTRATE: Kombucha House, Lot 7, Climax Court, Canaugra, Qld 4275. Tel: +61 75 435 104; Fax: +61 75 435 263.

HOMOEOPATHIC KOMBUCHA: Tina White, Manning Natural Healing Centre, 216 Victoria St, Taree, NSW 2430.

HOLLAND

SUPPLIES KOMBUCHA CULTURES/ BOOKS/ INFORMATION: Nelki Lauret, Lingedijk, 4001 XJ Tiel. Tel: 0344 612 956 Fax: 0344 614 517.

GERMANY

KOMBUCHA CULTURES: available from: **Günther Frank,** (Kombucha author) Genossenschafts Str.10, 75217 Birkenfeld im Schwartzwald, Germany.

READY BOTTLED KOMBUCHA/ KOMBUCHA DROPS: Dr Med Sklenar Bio-Produkte GMBH (Dr Sklenar Bio-Products), Mausegatt 8-12, D-4630 Bochum 6/Wattenscheid. Tel: 02327 10075.

READY BOTTLED KOMBUCHA TEA/HERBS/ GREEN TEA: Gerhard Kruger, Heilkrautervertrieb, Frankfurter Strasse 68, D-6338 Huttenberg OT Rechtenbach, Germany. Tel: 06441 74710.

SWITZERLAND

Dr Med Sklenar Bio-Produkte GMBH; Schweizerische Kombucha-Vertriebs-Zentrale (Swiss Kombucha Sales, Head Office), Postfach 135, CH-8600 Dubendorf, Zurich Orders accepted in writing only.
For information, Tel: 0155 69 71.

AUSTRIA

INFORMATION: Rosina Fasching (Kombucha author), PO Box 98, A-9021, Klagenfurt.

OTHER USEFUL ADDRESSES & PROFESSIONAL ASSOCIATIONS

EDUCATION

UK

Henry Doubleday Research Association
National Centre for Organic Gardening, Ryton-on-Dunsmore, Coventry, CV8 3LG
Demonstration organic gardens open to the public - research, information, garden supplies by mail order.

The Soil Association
86 Colston St., Bristol, BS1 5BB
Promotes all aspects of organic growing, nutrition, health and ecology; Vegetable and fruit growers and livestock farmers may apply for the Soil Association 'Symbol' which shows that food has been achieved through sustainable and humane methods. Under their 'Campaign for Safe Meat', the association produces a list of suppliers of organic meat including those who hold the Symbol.

The Good Gardeners Association (Int'l)
Pinetum Lodge, Churcham, Glos., GL2 8AD
Tel: 01452 750 402

Internet:
www.midnet.com/midnet.organic.gga
Information, newsletter, mail order. Organises conferences on all aspects of organic growing and good health.

Green Network
9 Clairmont Road, Lexdon, Colchester, Essex, CO3 5BE
Tel: 01206 46902; Fax: 01206 766 005
National organisation with international connections made up of individuals, organisations and businesses. Facilitates positive action for health and the environment. Network Magazine.

The Bristol Cancer Help Centre
Grove House, Cornwallis Grove, Clifton, Bristol, BS8 4PG
Tel: 0117 980 9500.
Patient Helpline: 0117 980 9505
An International Centre for the holistic approach to health for people with cancer and those who care for them. Residential and non-residential courses. Information - book and scientific database. Mail order - books, cassettes and video. Networks.

The Clouds Trust

38 Dennis Way,
Liss, Hants., GU33 7HL
Tel: 01730 301 162

A charity set up to research and supply the herbal tea known as the Rene Caisse formula (Essiac), and to establishing a retreat in the mountains above Nice for those with terminal illness.

Institute For Optimum Nutrition

Blades Court, Deodar Rd.,
London, SW15 2NU
Tel: 0181 877 9993; Fax: 0181 877 9980

Non-profit and independent organisation offering a variety of courses for the lay person and professionals (includes homestudy). Also consultations with qualified nutritionalists. Workshops, magazine, books, tapes and videos. Membership available.

Food For The Future

1 Eastfield Lane,
Whitchurch-on-Thames,
Nr Pangbourne, Oxon, RG8 7EJ
Tel: 0118 984 3303

A voluntary educational project in association with the Institute for Optimum Nutrition, whose aims are to inspire young people to take responsibility for their own health and for future generations.

Publishes health education material and teaching packages for schools. Informs; through training presenters, database, networking, news sheets and study days.

The Nutri Centre

7 Park Crescent
London, W1N 3HE
Tel: 0171 436 5122; Fax: 0171 436 5171

Bookshop and information on health issues.

The Myelin Trust (Multiple Sclerosis & Motor Nuerone Disease)

4 Cammo Walk,
Edinburgh, EH4 8AN

Tel: 0131 339 1316; Fax: 0131 317 1606

The National Osteoporosis Society

PO Box 10, Radstock,
Bath, Somerset, BA3 3YB
Tel: 01761 471 771; Fax: 01761 471 104
Helpline: 01761 472 721

USA

Rodale Research Center

RD Box 323, Kutztown, PA 18049

AUSTRALIA

Henry Doubleday Research Association of Australia

Box 61, Post Office,
Australia Square, NSW

SUPPLIERS

The Soil Association

Contact the Soil Association, address above; for a list of vegetable and livestock producers who adhere to the organic standards laid down by the Soil Association and who hold their 'Symbol'.

Nature's Own

Unit 8, Hanley Workshops
Hanley Rd., Hanley Swan,
Worcs, WR8 0DX
Tel: 01684 310 022; Fax: 01684 312 022

Highly recommended mail order vitamin and mineral supplements - includes 'Food State'.

G & G

175 London Rd, East Grinstead,
W. Sussex, RH19 1YY
Tel: 01342 312811; 24-hr: 01342 323016;
Fax: 01342 315938

Candida cleanse packs and supplements. Free advice line.

Hambledon Herbs

Court Farm, Milverton,
Somerset, TA4 1NF
Organic herb experts; culinary, spices and teas.

Sedlescoombe Vineyard

Cripps Corner, Nr Robertsbridge,
E. Sussex
Tel: 01580 830 715

Mail order organic English wines, juices and cider.

Bioflow Magnatherapy

Hamer Environment Leisure Products
805 Belmont Rd., Bolton,
Lancs, BL1 7BU
Tel: 01204 592 077

Mail order magnatherapy products; health-care for humans and animals.

ALTERNATIVE AND COMPLEMENTARY MEDICINE ORGANISATIONS

Send an s.a.e. for a list of registered practitioners:-

British College of Naturopathy and Osteopathy
6 Netherhall Gdns.,
London, NW3 5RR
Tel: 0171 435 7830

General Council and Register of Osteopaths
56 London St.,Reading,
Berks, RG1 4SQ
Tel: 01734 576 585

British Homoeopathic Association
27a Devonshire St.,
London, W1N 1RJ
Tel: 0171 935 2163

Bayly School of Reflexology
Monks Orchard, Whitbourne,
Worcs., WR6 5RB
Tel: 01886 821 207

British School of Shiatsu
6 Erskine Rd,
London, NW3 3AJ
0171 483 3776

Healing-Shiatsu Education Centre
The Orchard,
Lower-Maescoed,
Hereford, HR2 0HP
01873 860 207

International College of Oriental Medicine
Green Hedges House,
Green Hedges Ave.,
East Grinstead, W. Sussex, RH19 1DZ
Tel: 01342 313 106/7

British Wheel of Yoga
1 Hamilton Pl., Boston Rd.,
Sleaford, Lincs., NG34 7ES
Tel: 01529 306 851

National Institute of Medical Herbalists
9 Palace Gate,
Exeter, EX1 1JA
Tel: 01392 426 022

Aromatherapy Organisation Council
3 Latymer Close, Braybrook,
Market Harborough,
Leics., LE16 8LN
Tel: 01858 434 242

Society of Teachers of The Alexander Technique
20 London House,
266 Fulham Rd.,
London, SW10 9EL
Tel: 0171 351 0828

World Federation of Spiritual Healers
Mr Lyonel Thomas,
8 Earl Rd., Penarth,
So.Glam., CF64 3UN
Tel: 01222 703 640

INDEX

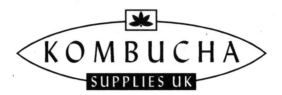

KOMBUCHA
SUPPLIES UK

The Hollies, Mill Hill, Wellow, Bath, BA2 8QJ, UK

Telephone: 01225 833 150 (Overseas: 44 1225 833 150)
Fax: 01225 840 012 (Overseas: 44 1225 840 012)

FOR ALL YOUR KOMBUCHA BREWING NEEDS

Kombucha Electric Heating Trays

Provides low wattage controlled heat, giving the ideal constant liquid temperature for Kombucha brewing. Four sizes. Two year guarantee. Available with standard U.K. voltage and plug, or can be supplied for USA and Continental Europe.

pH Test Strips

The acidity or pH level of the fermenting Kombucha tea can be tested correctly with these inexpensive test strips.

Kombucha Cream

This 'live' Kombucha cream is made from all natural ingredients (without animal derivatives), and is suitable for many skin complaints and for massage.

Kombucha Capsules

Made from dried extract of the Kombucha liquid. Ideal for travelling, or if you are unable to brew you own Kombucha tea.

Digital Strip Thermometer

Used to determine the ideal temperature for your Kombucha fermentation. Inexpensive and recommended.

Chinese Green Tea

Well documented and researched as containing anti-carcinogenic properties and also as benefical for the heart. An extra bonus is that it makes a lovely light, fresh, 'zingy' Kombucha tea.

Paw Paw Concentrate and the Rene Caisse Formula Herbal Tea

(also known as Essiac) Either or both of these herbal/fruit preparations taken in combination with Kombucha tea have given significant results for people with cancer.

We sell Kombucha books and a range of other health-related books and audio tapes.

We also provide a Kombucha advice line on weekday mornings.

Wishing you good health!

PLEASE CONTACT US FOR A FREE CATALOGUE